W9-DDH-265

# The Orange Man

# The Orange Man

## And Other Narratives of
## Medical Detection

by Berton Roueché

BOSTON • LITTLE, BROWN AND COMPANY • TORONTO

COPYRIGHT © 1965, 1966, 1967, 1968, 1969, 1970, 1971
BY BERTON ROUECHÉ

ALL RIGHTS RESERVED. NO PART OF THIS BOOK MAY BE REPRODUCED
IN ANY FORM OR BY ANY ELECTRONIC OR MECHANICAL MEANS IN-
CLUDING INFORMATION STORAGE AND RETRIEVAL SYSTEMS WITHOUT
PERMISSION IN WRITING FROM THE PUBLISHER, EXCEPT BY A REVIEWER
WHO MAY QUOTE BRIEF PASSAGES IN A REVIEW.

LIBRARY OF CONGRESS CATALOG CARD NO. 70-160696
TO 9/71
FIRST EDITION

The stories that compose this book
first appeared in *The New Yorker*

*Published simultaneously in Canada
by Little, Brown & Company (Canada) Limited*

PRINTED IN THE UNITED STATES OF AMERICA

*For Gardner Botsford*

We have more effectively eliminated the buffalo,
the whooping crane, and the trailing arbutus
than we have obliterated the causes of disease.
Thomas Francis, Jr., M.D. (1900–1969)

# Contents

# The Orange Man

# The Orange Man

Around eleven-thirty on the morning of December 15, 1960, Dr. Richard L. Wooten, an internist and an assistant professor of internal medicine at the University of Tennessee College of Medicine, in Memphis, was informed by the receptionist in the office he shares with several associates that a patient named (I'll say) Elmo Turner was waiting to see him. Dr. Wooten remembered Turner, but not much about him. He asked the receptionist to fetch him Turner's folder, and then, when she had done so, to send Turner right on in. The folder refreshed his memory. Turner was fifty-three years old, married, and a plumber by trade, and over the past ten years Dr. Wooten had seen him through an attack of pneumonia and referred him along for treatment of a variety of troubles, including a fractured wrist and a hip-joint condition. There

3

were footsteps in the hall. Dr. Wooten closed the folder. The door opened, and Turner — a short, thick, muscular man — came in. Dr. Wooten had risen to greet him, but for a moment he could only stand and stare. Turner's face was orange — a golden, pumpkin orange. So were both his hands.

Dr. Wooten found his voice. He gave Turner a friendly good morning, asked him to sit down, and remarked that it had been a couple of years since their last meeting. Turner agreed that it had. He had been away. He had been working up in Alaska — in Fairbanks. He and his wife were back in Memphis only on a matter of family business. But, being in town, he thought he ought to pay Dr. Wooten a visit. There was something that kind of bothered him. Dr. Wooten listened with half an ear. His mind was searching through the spectrum of pathological skin discolorations. There were many diseases with pigmentary manifestations. There was the paper pallor of pituitary disease. There was the cyanotic blue of congenital heart disease. There was the deep Florida tan of thyroid dysfunction. There was the jaundice yellow of liver damage. There was the bronze of hemochromatosis. As far as he knew, however, there was no disease that colored its victims orange. Turner's voice recalled him. In fact, he was saying, he was worried. Dr. Wooten nodded. Just what seemed to be the trouble? Turner touched his abdomen with a bright-orange hand. He had a pain down there. His abdomen had been sore off and on for over a year, but now it was more than sore. It hurt. Dr. Wooten gave an encouraging grunt, and waited. He waited for Turner to say something about his extraordinary color. But Turner had finished. He had said all he had to say. Apparently, it was only his abdomen that worried him.

Dr. Wooten stood up. He asked Turner to come along

down the hall to the examining room. His color, however bizarre, could wait. A chronic abdominal pain came first. And not only that. The cause of Turner's pain was probably also the cause of his color. That seemed, at least, a reasonable assumption. They entered the examining room. Dr. Wooten switched on the light above the examination table and turned and looked at Turner. The light in his office had been an ordinary electric light, and ordinary electric light has a faintly yellow tinge. The examining room had a true-color daylight light. But Turner's color owed nothing to tricks of light. His skin was still an unearthly golden orange. Turner stripped to the waist and got up on the table and stretched out on his back. His torso was as orange as his face. Dr. Wooten began his examination. He found the painful abdominal area, and carefully pressed. There was something there. He could feel an abnormality — a deep-seated mass about the size of an apple. It was below and behind the stomach, and he thought it might be sited at the liver. He pressed again. It wasn't the liver. It was positioned too near the center of the stomach for that. It was the pancreas.

Dr. Wooten moved away from the table. He had learned all he could from manual exploration. He waited for Turner to dress, and then led the way back to his office. He told Turner what he had found. He said he couldn't identify the mass he had felt, and he wouldn't attempt to guess. Its nature could be determined only by a series of X-ray examinations. That, he was sorry to say, would require a couple of days in the hospital. The pancreas was seated too deep to be accessible to direct X-ray examination, and an indirect examination took time and special preparation. Turner listened, and shrugged. He was willing to do whatever had to be done. Dr. Wooten swiveled

5

around in his chair and picked up the telephone. He put in a call to the admitting office of Baptist Memorial Hospital, an affiliate of the medical school, and had a few words with the reservations clerk. He swiveled back to Turner. It was all arranged. Turner would be expected at Baptist Memorial at three o'clock that afternoon. Turner nodded, and got up to go. Dr. Wooten waved him back into his chair. There was one more thing. It was about the color of his skin. How long had it been like that? Turner looked blank. Color? What color? What was wrong with the color of his skin. Dr. Wooten hesitated. He was startled. There was no mistaking Turner's reaction. He was genuinely confused. He didn't know about his color — he really didn't know. And that was an interesting thought. It was, in fact, instructive. It clearly meant that Turner's change of color was not a sudden development. It had come on slowly, insidiously, imperceptibly. He realized that Turner was waiting, that his question had to be answered. Dr. Wooten answered it. Turner looked even blanker. He gazed at his hands, and then at Dr. Wooten. He didn't see anything unusual about his color. His skin was naturally ruddy. It always looked this way.

Dr. Wooten let it go at that. There was no point in pressing the matter any further right then. It would only worry Turner, and he was worried enough already. The matter would keep until the afternoon, until the next day, until he had a little more information to work with. He leaned back and lighted a cigarette, and changed the subject. Or seemed to. Had Turner ever met the senior associate here? That was Dr. Hughes — Dr. John D. Hughes. No? Well, in that case . . . Dr. Wooten reached for the telephone. Dr. Hughes's office was just next door, and he arrived a moment later. He walked into the room and glanced at Turner, and stopped — and stared. Dr. Wooten introduced them. He described the reason for Turner's visit and the mass he had found in the region of the pancreas. Dr. Hughes subdued his stare to a look of polite attention. They talked for several minutes. When Turner got up again to go, Dr. Wooten saw him to the door. He came back to his desk and sat down. Well, what did Dr. Hughes make of that? Had he ever seen or read or even heard of a man that color before? Dr. Hughes said no. And he didn't know what to think. He was completely flabbergasted. He was rather uneasy, too. That, Dr. Wooten said, made two of them.

Turner was admitted to Baptist Memorial Hospital for observation that afternoon at a few minutes after three. He was given the usual admission examination and assigned a bed in a ward. An hour or two later, Dr. Wooten, in the course of his regular hospital rounds, stopped by Turner's bed for the ritual visit of welcome and reassurance. Turner appeared to be no more than reasonably nervous, and Dr. Wooten found that satisfactory. He then turned his attention to Turner's chart and the results of the admission examination. They were, as expected, unrevealing. Turner's temperature was normal. So were his pulse rate (seventy-eight beats a minute), his respiration rate (sixteen respirations a minute), and his blood pressure (a hundred and ten systolic, eighty diastolic). The results of the urinalysis and of an electrocardiographic examination were also normal. Before resuming his rounds, Dr. Wooten satisfied himself that the really important examinations had been scheduled. These were comprehensive X-ray studies of

7

the chest, upper gastrointestinal tract, and colon. The first two examinations were down for the following morning.

They were made at about eight o'clock. When Dr. Wooten reached the hospital on a midmorning tour, the radiologist's report was in and waiting. It more than confirmed Dr. Wooten's impression of the location of the mass. It defined its nature as well. The report read, "Lung fields are clear. Heart is normal. Barium readily traversed the esophagus and entered the stomach. In certain positions, supine projections, an apparent defect was seen on the stomach. However, this was extrinsic to the stomach. It may well represent a pseudocyst of the pancreas. No lesions of the stomach itself were demonstrated. Duodenal bulb and loop appeared normal. Stomach was emptying in a satisfactory manner." Dr. Wooten put down the report with a shiver of relief. A pancreatic cyst — even a pseudocyst — is not a trifling affliction, but he welcomed that diagnosis. The mass on Turner's pancreas just might have been a tumor. It hadn't been a likely possibility — the mass was too large and the symptoms were too mild — but it had been a possibility.

Dr. Wooten went up to Turner's ward. He told Turner what the X-ray examination had shown and what the findings meant. A cyst was a sac retaining a liquid normally excreted by the body. A pseudocyst was an empty sac — a mere dilation of space. The only known treatment of a pancreatic cyst was surgical, and surgery involving the pancreas was difficult and dangerous. Surgery was difficult because of the remote location of the pancreas, and dangerous because of the delicacy of the organs surrounding the pancreas (the stomach, the spleen, the duodenum) and the delicacy of the functions of the pancreas (the production of enzymes essential to digestion and

8

the secretion of insulin). Fortunately, however, treatment was seldom necessary. Most cysts — particularly pseudocysts — had a way of disappearing as mysteriously as they had come. It was his belief that this was such a cyst. In that case, there was nothing much to do but be patient. And careful. Turner was to guard his belly from sudden bumps or strains. A blow or a wrench could cause a lot of trouble.

Nevertheless, Dr. Wooten went on, he wanted Turner to remain in the hospital for at least another day. There was a final X-ray of the colon to be made, and several other tests. In view of this morning's findings, the examination was, he admitted, very largely a matter of form. The cause of Turner's abdominal pain was definitely a pseudocyst of the pancreas. But prudence required an X-ray, and it would probably be done the next day. It was usual, for technical reasons, to let a day elapse between an upper-gastrointestinal study and a colon examination. Two of the other tests were indicated by the X-ray findings. One was a test for diabetes — the glucose-tolerance test. Diabetes was a possible complication of a cyst of the pancreas. Pressure from the cyst could produce diabetes by disrupting the production of insulin in the pancreatic islets of Langerhans. Such pressure could also cause another complication — a blockage of the common bile duct. The diagnostic test for that was a chemical analysis of the blood serum for the presence of the bile pigment known as bilirubin. Dr. Wooten paused. The time had come to reopen the subject that he had tactfully dropped the day before. He reopened it. It was possible, he said, that the bilirubin test might help explain the unusual color of Turner's skin. And Turner's skin *was* a most unusual color. He held up an adamant hand. No. Turner was mistaken. His color *had* changed in the past year or two. It wasn't a natural

9

ruddiness. It was a highly unnatural orange. It was a sign that something was wrong, and he intended to find out what. That was the reason for a third test he had ordered. It was a diagnostic blood test for a condition called hemochromatosis. Hemochromatosis was a disturbance of iron metabolism that deposited iron in the skin and stained it the color of bronze. To be frank, he didn't hope for much from either of the pigmentation tests. Turner's color wasn't the bronze of hemochromatosis, and it wasn't the yellow of jaundice. The possibility of jaundice was particularly remote. The whites of Turner's eyes were still white, and that was usually where jaundice made its first appearance. But he had to carry out the tests. He had to be sure. The process of elimination was always an instructive process. And they didn't have long to wait. The results of the tests would be ready sometime that afternoon. He would be back to see Turner then.

Dr. Wooten spent the next few hours at the hospital and his office. He had other patients to see, other problems to consider, other decisions to make. But Turner remained on his mind. His first impression, like so many first impressions, had been mistaken. It now seemed practically certain that Turner's color had no connection with Turner's pancreatic cyst. They were two quite different complaints. And that returned him to the question he had asked himself when Turner walked into his office. What did an orange skin signify? What disease had the power to turn its victims orange? The answer, as before, was none. But perhaps this wasn't in the usual sense a disease. Perhaps it was a drug-induced reaction. Many chemicals in common therapeutic and diagnostic use were capable of producing conspicuous skin discolorations. Or it might be related to diet.

The question hung in Dr. Wooten's mind all day. It was still hanging there when he headed back to Turner's ward. On the way, he picked up the results of the tests he had ordered that morning, and they did nothing to resolve it. Turner's total bilirubin level was 0.9 milligrams per hundred milliliters, or normal. The total iron-binding capacity was also normal — 286 micrograms per hundred milliliters. And he didn't have diabetes. When Dr. Wooten came into the ward, he found Turner's wife at his bedside and Turner in a somewhat altered state of mind. He said he had begun to think that maybe Dr. Wooten was right about the color of his skin. There must be something peculiar about it. There had been a parade of doctors and nurses past his bed ever since early morning. Mrs. Turner looked bewildered. She hadn't noticed anything unusual about her husband's color. She hadn't thought about it — the question had never come up. But now that it had, she had to admit that he did look kind of different. He did look kind of orange. But what was the reason? What in the world could cause a thing like that? Dr. Wooten said he didn't know. The most he could say at the moment was that certain possibilities had been eliminated. He summarized the results of the three diagnostic tests. Another possible cause, he then went on to say, was drugs. Medicinal drugs. Certain medicines incorporated dyes or chemicals with pigmentary properties. Turner shook his head. Maybe so, he said, but that was out. It had been months since he had taken any kind of drug except aspirin.

Dr. Wooten was glad to believe him. Drugs had been a rather farfetched possibility. The color changes they produced were generally dramatically sudden and almost never lasting. He turned to another area — to diet. What did Turner like to eat? What, for example, did he usually have for breakfast? That was no problem, Turner said. His breakfast was almost always the same — orange juice, bacon and eggs, toast, coffee. And what about lunch? Well, that didn't change much, either. He ate a lot of vegetables — carrots, rutabagas, squash, beans, spinach, turnips, things like that. Mrs. Turner laughed. That, she said, was putting it mildly. He ate carrots the way some people eat candy. Dr. Wooten sat erect. Carrots, he was abruptly aware, were rich in carotene. So were eggs, oranges, rutabagas, squash, beans, spinach, and turnips. And carotene was a powerful yellow pigment. What, he asked Mrs. Turner, did she mean about the way her husband ate carrots? Mrs. Turner laughed again. She meant just what she said. Elmo was always eating carrots. Eating carrots and drinking tomato juice. Tomato juice was his favorite drink. And carrots were his favorite snack. He ate raw carrots all day long. He ate four or five of them a day. Why, driving down home from Alaska last week, he kept her busy just scraping and slicing and feeding him carrots. Turner gave an embarrassed grin. His wife was right. He reckoned he did eat a lot of carrots. But he had his reasons. You needed extra vitamins when you lived in Alaska. You had to make up for the long, dark winters — the lack of sunlight up there. Dr. Wooten stood up to go. What the Turners had told him was extremely interesting. He was sure, he said, that Turner's appetite for carrots was a clue to the cause of his color. It was also, as it happened, misguided. The so-called "sunshine vitamin" was Vitamin D. The vitamin with which carrots and other yellow vegetables were abundantly endowed was Vitamin A.

There was a telephone just down the hall from Turner's ward. Dr. Wooten stopped and put in a call to the hospital laboratory. He arranged with the technician who took the call for a sample of Turner's blood to be tested for an abnormal concentration of carotene. Then he left the hospital and cut across the campus to the Mooney Memorial Library. He asked the librarian to let him see what she could find in the way of clinical literature on carotenemia and any related nutritional skin discolorations. He was elated by what he had learned from the Turners, but he knew that it wasn't enough. He had seen several cases of carotenemia. An excessive intake of carotene was a not uncommon condition among health-bar habitués and other amateur nutritionists. But carotene didn't color people orange. It colored them yellow. Or such had been his experience.

The librarian reported that papers on carotenemia were scarce. She had, however, found three clinical studies that looked as though they might be useful. Here was one of them. She handed Dr. Wooten a bound volume of the *Journal of the American Medical Association* for 1919, and indicated the relevant article. It was a report by two New York City investigators — Alfred F. Hess and Victor C. Myers — entitled "Carotinemia: A New Clinical Picture." Dr. Wooten knew their report, at least by reputation. It was the original study in the field. The opening descriptive paragraphs refreshed his memory and confirmed his judgment. They read:

About a year ago one of us (A.F.H.) observed that two children in a ward containing about twenty-five infants, from a year to a year and a half in age, were developing a yellowish complexion. This coloration was not confined to the face, but involved, to a less extent, the entire body, being most evident on the palms of the hands. . . . For a time, we were at a loss to account for this peculiar phenomenon, when our attention was directed to the fact that these two children, and only these two, were receiving a

13

daily ration of carrots in addition to their milk and cereal. For some time we had been testing the food value of dehydrated vegetables, and when the change in color was noted, had given these babies the equivalent of 2 tablespoonfuls of fresh carrots for a period of six weeks.

It seemed as if this mild jaundiced hue might well be the result of the introduction into the body of a pigment rather than the manifestation of a pathologic condition. Attention was accordingly directed to the carrots, and the same amount of this vegetable was added to the dietary of two other children of about the same age. In the one instance, after an interval of about five weeks, a yellowish tinge of the skin was noted, and about two weeks later the other baby had become somewhat yellow. There was a decided difference in the intensity of color of the four infants, indicating probably that the alteration was in part governed by individual idiosyncrasy. On omission of the carrots from the dietary, the skin gradually lost its yellow color, and in the course of some weeks regained its normal tint.

The librarian returned to Dr. Wooten's table with the other references. Both were contributions to the *New England Journal of Medicine*. One was entitled "Skin Changes of Nutritional Origin," and had been written by Harold Jeghers, an associate professor of medicine at the Boston University School of Medicine, in 1943. The other was the work of three faculty members of the Harvard Medical School — Peter Reich, Harry Shwachman, and John M. Craig — and was entitled "Lycopenemia: A Variant of Carotenemia." It had appeared in 1960. Dr. Wooten looked first at "Skin Changes of Nutritional Origin." It was a comprehensive survey, and it read, in part:

The carotenoid group of pigments color the serum and fix themselves to the fat of the dermis and subcutaneous tissues, to which they impart the yellow tint. . . . Edwards and Duntley showed by means of spectrophotometric analysis of skin color in human beings that carotene is present in every normal skin and is one of the five basic pigments that determine the skin color of every living person. Clinically, therefore, carotenemia refers to the presence of an excess over normal of carotene in the skin and serum. . . . In most cases carotenemia results simply from excess use of foods rich in the carotenoid pigments. Individuals probably vary in the ease with which carotenemia develops, which is evidenced by the fact that many vegetarians do not develop it. It is said to develop more readily in those who sweat profusely. Except for the yellow color produced, it appears to be harmless, even though present for months. It eventually disappears over several weeks to months when the carotene consumption is reduced.

Dr. Wooten moved on to the third report. ("This investigation concerns a middle-aged woman whose prolonged and excessive consumption of tomato juice led to the discoloration of her skin.") He read it slowly through from beginning to end, and then turned back and reread certain passages:

Although carotenemia due to the ingestion of foods containing a high concentration of beta carotene is a commonly described disorder, a similar condition secondary to the ingestion of tomatoes and associated with high serum levels of lycopene has not previously been reported. . . . Lycopene is a common carotenoid pigment widely distributed through nature. It is most familiar as the red pigment of tomatoes, but has been detected in many animals and vegetables. . . . It is also frequently found in human serum and liver, especially when tomatoes are eaten. But lycopene is not well known medically because, unlike beta carotene, it is physiologically inert and has not been involved in any form of illness.

Dr. Wooten closed the volume. Turner was not only a heavy eater of carrots. He was also a heavy drinker of tomato juice. Carrots are rich in carotene and tomatoes are rich in lycopene. Carotene is a yellow pigment and lycopene is red. And yellow and red make orange.

Dr. Wooten completed his record of the case with a double

diagnosis: pseudocyst of the pancreas and carotenemia-lycopenemia. The results of the X-ray examination of Turner's colon were normal ("Terminal ileum was visualized. No pathology was demonstrated in the colon"), and the carotene test showed a high concentration of serum carotenoids (495 micrometers per hundred milliliters, compared to a normal concentration of 50 to 350 micrometers per hundred milliliters). The diagnosis of lycopenemia was made from the clinical evidence. Turner was discharged from the hospital on December 17. His instructions were to avoid abdominal blows, carrots (and other yellow vegetables), and tomatoes in any form. Four months later, on April 16, 1961, he reported to Dr. Wooten that his skin had recovered its normal ruddiness. Two years later, in 1963, he returned again to Memphis and dropped in on Dr. Wooten for a visit. His abdominal symptoms had long since disappeared, and a comprehensive examination showed no sign of the pseudocyst.

Elmo Turner was the first recorded victim of the condition known as carotenemia-lycopenemia. He is not, however, the only one now on record. Another victim turned up in 1964. She was a woman of thirty-five, a resident of Memphis, and a patient of Dr. Wooten's. He had been treating her for a mild diabetes since 1962, and had put her at that time on the eighteen-hundred-calorie diet recommended by the American Diabetes Association. She had faithfully followed the diet, but in order to do so had eaten heavily of low-calorie vegetables, and (as she confirmed, with some surprise, when questioned) the vegetables she ate most heavily were carrots and tomatoes. She ate at least two cups of carrots and at least two whole tomatoes every day. Dr. Wooten was unaware of this until she walked into his office one October day in 1964 for her semi-annual consultation. He greeted her as calmly as he could, and asked her to sit down. He would be back in just a moment. He stepped along the hall to Dr. Hughes's office and looked in. Dr. Hughes was alone.

"Have you got a minute, John?" Dr. Wooten said.

"Sure," Dr. Hughes said. "What is it?"

"I'd like you to come into my office," Dr. Wooten said. "I'd like to show you something."

# Three Sick Babies

$\text{D}$r. Paul M. Taylor, an assistant professor of pediatrics
at the University of Pittsburgh School of Medicine, left his
office on the first floor of Magee-Womens Hospital, an affiliate
of the medical school, and climbed the stairs to the premature-
baby nursery, on the second floor. It was twenty minutes to
eleven on the morning of July 12, 1965, a Monday, and this
was his regular weekday round. He was, in a way, attending
physician to all the babies in the nursery. Two pediatric residents were waiting for him in the gown room. That, too, was
as usual, and while Dr. Taylor scrubbed and disinfected his
hands and got into a freshly laundered gown, they gave him
the customary nursery news report. The weekend had been
generally uneventful. All but one of the twenty-six babies in
the nursery were progressing satisfactorily. The exception was

quickly controlled with penicillin, kanamycin, and dexamethasone. His trouble now was diarrhea. Diarrhea in a newborn baby is not a common complaint, and Dr. Taylor wondered if this attack might be a septic aftermath of the earlier pneumonia. But that was a question that only the laboratory could readily answer. There was no doubt about the treatment the baby was receiving. That seemed to be entirely satisfactory.

The Wednesday-morning gown-room news review contained three major items. One was that still another baby boy had become seriously ill overnight. The next item was a preliminary laboratory report on the second sick baby, which identified the cause of his diarrhea as a gram-negative bacillus. The third item was a more or less definitive laboratory report on the dead baby. After forty-eight hours of growth, the gram-negative bacteria cultured from his blood presented the colonial configuration, the fluorescent yellow-green pigmentation, and the spearmint odor generally characteristic of the type known as Pseudomonas aeruginosa.

Dr. Taylor went to Room 229 for a look at the new sick boy. He was nine days old and weighed about three pounds. His illness appeared to be a pneumonia. This illness had come abruptly, but, like so many other premature babies, he had never been really well. He had been unable at birth to breathe spontaneously and had spent the first five or six days of his life in a respirator. It was obvious to Dr. Taylor that the baby's condition was grave. It seemed equally clear, however, that he was receiving the best of care, and a conventional course of penicillin and kanamycin had been started. Dr. Taylor left the nursery in an uneasy state of mind. His uneasiness had to do with Room 229 and the sudden string of serious illnesses there.

one of the smallest — a twenty-five-day-old two-and-a-half-pound boy. He was in Room 227. Dr. Taylor nodded. He knew the one they meant. Well, early that morning, just after midnight, a nurse had noted that his breathing was unusually slow and his behavior somewhat apathetic. The resident on duty, seeing these signs as suggestive of septicemia, had treated the baby with penicillin and kanamycin, but he still looked and acted sick. It was probable that he would soon need artificial respiration. Meanwhile, the usual samples (blood, stool, mucus, spinal fluid) had been taken and sent along to the laboratory for culture and analysis.

Dr. Taylor heard his residents' review with no more than natural interest. Serious illness in a premature nursery is not an unusual occurrence, and a blood infection is only one of the many diseases that may afflict a premature baby during its first days of life. Trouble is inherent in the phenomenon of prematurity. For the truth of the matter is that premature birth is itself a serious affliction. A premature baby is a baby born in the seventh or eighth month of pregnancy. Its birth weight is largely determined by its relative prematurity, ranging from around two to five and a half pounds. The average term (or nine-month) baby weighs around seven pounds at birth, and it generally comes into the world alive and kicking. Premature babies begin life almost incapable of living. There is nothing more frail and fragile. Many of them are too meagerly developed to maintain normal body temperature. One in three requires immediate, and often prolonged, resuscitation, and about the same number are unable to nurse, or even to swallow. Some of them are even unable to cry. All of them are exquisitely susceptible to all infection. Mental and neurological defects are also common in premature babies. One of the commonest of these is cerebral palsy. About half of all victims of the affliction are of premature birth. As recently as twenty-five years ago, most premature babies died. The technological innovations of the postwar era have greatly improved that record, but the mortality rate among newborn premature babies is still high. In even the best hospitals, some ninety percent of all two-pound babies die. So do about fifty percent of those weighing two to three pounds, around ten percent of those weighing three to four pounds, and between five and eight percent of those weighing four to five pounds. Such babies are simply too fetal to survive outside the womb. There are many causes of premature birth (including falls and blows), but most current investigators think that malnutrition is perhaps the most important cause. Prematurity would thus seem to be a socioeconomic problem, and this supposition is confirmed by statistics. The great majority of premature babies are born to women too poor to buy the nutritious food they need.

Dr. Taylor tied up the back of his gown and led the way through an inner door to the central nursing station of the nursery. Room 227 was the second room on the right. The sick baby was one of five babies being cared for there. He lay on his side in his incubator bassinet with a stomach feeding tube in his mouth, and he looked even sicker than the resident had said. There was nothing, however, that Dr. Taylor could do that hadn't already been done. He confirmed the resident's course of treatment and agreed that a respirator would probably soon be required, and then moved on to the other babies in that and the other rooms. They were all, as far as he could read the almost imperceptible manifestations of the premature, in their usual precarious but normal condition. At the end of

his rounds, Dr. Taylor had lunch, and after lunch[ ]himself with his other professorial duties. Befor[ ]home, he put in a call to the nursery for a repo[ ]baby. The report was not comforting. The ba[ ]had continued to worsen, and he had been m[ ]229, which is reserved for babies needing const[ ]care. Later that evening, on his way to bed,[ ]nursery again. The nurse who picked up the[ ]able to answer his question. The sick baby from[ ]dead.

Dr. Taylor's Tuesday-morning round was n[ ]Monday. The residents' gown-room report i[ ]sick baby. It also contained a post-mortem n[ ]from Room 227. The hospital laboratory ha[ ]general diagnosis of septicemia. A microbial[ ]grown from a sample of the baby's blood[ ]bacteria of the gram-negative type. It was on[ ]five species of bacteria (among them the c[ ]of typhoid fever, brucellosis, whooping c[ ]gonorrhea) that react negatively to the sta[ ]devised in 1884 by the Danish bacteriolog[ ]Joachim Gram. A more specific identifica[ ]for the next day. Meanwhile, of course,[ ]been supplied with diagnostic samples fr[ ]baby. This baby, also a boy, was one of[ ]229. He was a term baby, three days old, b[ ]to the premature nursery directly from[ ]because he required artificial respiration[ ]care. Dr. Taylor remembered the baby v[ ]had begun life with a severe aspiration[ ]from an original inability to breathe,

He was afraid that they might be more than merely coincidental.

Dr. Taylor was not kept in suspense for long. One of his fears was confirmed that afternoon by a call from the resident then on duty in the nursery. He called to report that the new sick baby — the three-pound nine-day-old — was dead. His illness had lasted a scant eight hours. The next morning brought another confirmation. There was a final laboratory report on the first sick baby: the cause of his death was definitely a Pseudomonas infection. There was a forty-eight-hour report on the second sick baby: the gram-negative bacteria grown from his blood had all the important characteristics of Pseudomonas aeruginosa. There was a twenty-four-hour report on the third sick baby: cultures grown from his blood had been identified as gram-negative bacteria. And that was too much for coincidence. It meant — it could almost certainly only mean — that a Pseudomonas epidemic had struck the premature nursery.

Pseudomonas aeruginosa is one of a group of gram-negative pathogens that have only recently come to be seriously pathogenic. Other members of this group include Escherichia coli and the several species of the Proteus and the Enterobacter-Klebsiella genera. Their rise to eminent virulence is a curious phenomenon. These microorganisms regularly reside in soil and water, and in the gastrointestinal tracts of most (if not all) human beings. Their presence in that part of the body is normally innocuous. Healthy adults are impervious to the thrust of such bacteria. The victims of Pseudomonas (and E. coli and Proteus and Enterobacter) infections are the very old, the

23

very young, and the very debilitated (the badly burned, the postoperative, the cancerous), and in almost every case they have been receiving vigorous sulfonamide or antibiotic or adrenalsteroid therapy. Most antimicrobial drugs have little destructive effect on bacteria of the Pseudomonas group. Just the reverse, in fact. Their action, in essence, is tonic. In people rendered susceptible to the gram-negative pathogens by age or illness, the result of chemotherapy is the elimination not only of the immediately threatening pathogens but also of the natural resident bacteria that normally hold further incursions of Pseudomonas (or E. coli or Proteus or Enterobacter) in check. The virulence of Pseudomonas and its kind is thus a wry expression of perhaps the most beneficent accomplishment of twentieth-century medicine.

It is also cause for some alarm. "One of the great changes wrought by the widespread use of antibacterial agents has been the radical shift in the ecologic relations among the pathogenic bacteria that are responsible for the most serious and fatal infections," the *New England Journal of Medicine* noted editorially in July of 1967. "Whereas John Bunyan could properly refer to consumption as 'Captain of the Men of Death,' this title, according to Osler, was taken over by pneumonia in the first quarter of this century. During the last two decades, it has again shifted, at least in hospital populations, first to the staphylococcal diseases and more recently to infections caused by gram-negative bacilli. Most of the gram-negative organisms that have given rise to these serious and highly fatal infections are among the normal flora of the bowel and have sometimes been referred to as 'opportunistic pathogens.' . . . Before the present antibiotic era, some of them, like Escherichia coli, although they frequently caused simple urinary-tract infections,

24

only occasionally gave rise to serious sepsis. . . . Strains of Proteus or Pseudomonas did so very rarely, and those of Enterobacter were not even known to produce infections in human beings before the introduction of sulfonamide drugs. Of great importance are the facts that most of these opportunistic pathogens are resistant to the antibiotics that have been most widely used, and that the infections they produce are associated with a high mortality." This mortality is anachronistically high. It is roughly that resulting from the common run of pathogenic bacteria some thirty years ago — in the days when the best defense against the many Men of Death was a strong constitution.

The most conspicuously troublesome of these ordinarily unaggressive pathogens is E. coli. It has been implicated in some ninety percent of the urinary-tract infections caused by members of this group, and it is responsible for many of the more serious cases of bacteremia, gastroenteritis, and pneumonia. It is not, however, the most opportunistic. The organism best equipped to take advantage of almost any chemotherapeutic opportunity is the Pseudomonas bacillus. Pseudomonas aeruginosa is all but invulnerable to the present pharmacopoeia. Only two antibiotics — polymyxin B and colistin — are generally effective against most Pseudomonas strains. Moreover, both must be used with great discretion to prevent severe kidney side reactions. Ps. aeruginosa is also distinctively lethal. Its mortality rate, as numerous recent outbreaks (including that in Pittsburgh in 1965) have shown, may run as high as seventy-five percent.

An investigation into the source of the Pseudomonas infections in the premature nursery at Magee-Womens Hospital was started by Dr. Taylor on Friday morning, July 16. A forty-eight-hour report from the laboratory had by then established as Ps. aeruginosa the gram-negative bacteria that had been cultured from the blood of the third sick baby, and the presence of an epidemic was now beyond dispute. The investigation began with a survey to determine the scope of the trouble. There were at that time, in addition to the surviving (or diarrheal) sick baby, twenty-eight babies in the nursery. Samples of nose, throat, and stool material were taken from each, to be dispatched to the laboratory for culture and analysis. Dr. Taylor saw this work well under way, and then walked down to his office and put in a call to a colleague named Horace M. Gezon, at the Graduate School of Public Health. Dr. Gezon (at the time professor of epidemiology and microbiology at the University of Pittsburgh Graduate School of Public Health and now chairman of the Department of Pediatrics at the Boston University School of Medicine) is an authority on hospital infections, and Dr. Taylor wanted his help. Dr. Gezon had two immediate suggestions. One was that the investigators meet at the hospital the following morning for an exchange of information and ideas. The other was that Joshua Fierer, of the Allegheny County Health Department, be invited to join the investigation. Dr. Fierer (now a postdoctoral fellow in infectious diseases at the University of Pittsburgh Department of Medicine) was an Epidemic Intelligence Service officer assigned to Allegheny County by the National Communicable Disease Center, in Atlanta.

"Dr. Taylor called me on Friday afternoon," Dr. Fierer says. "I know it was Friday, because that's when all investigations seem to begin — at the start of the weekend. I knew Dr. Taylor. I had met him with Dr. Gezon back in March — on a Friday in March. There had been an outbreak of diarrhea in the premature nursery that they thought might be a viral disease, and they called the county because we had the only virus-diagnostic laboratory in the area. That case turned out to be nothing to worry about. It got the three of us together, though, and I guess that was what brought me to mind when this new problem came up. I was delighted to be asked to participate. Pseudomonas is a very interesting organism these days. But I had to tell Dr. Taylor that I couldn't make the Saturday-morning meeting. Or, if I could, I'd be late. I had a firm commitment at the Pittsburgh Children's Zoo on Saturday morning. They had a chimpanzee out there with hepatitis.

"I got to the hospital, but I was more than late. It was after lunch, and the meeting was over and everybody had gone. I looked around the nursery, feeling kind of foolish, and said hello to the nurses, and they told me who had been at the meeting. There were six in the group, including Dr. Taylor and Dr. Gezon. The others were the two residents, a study nurse of Dr. Gezon's, and an assistant professor of epidemiology at the School of Public Health named Russell Rycheck. Dr. Rycheck was a particular friend of mine. I went over to the school and looked him up, and he gave me a good report. The meeting had naturally concentrated on the nursery. The big question, of course, was: Where had the infection come from? How had Pseudomonas been introduced into the nursery? Well, Pseudomonas is a water-dwelling organism. It can live on practically nothing in the merest drop of water. That suggested water as the probable source of the trouble, and the nursery had plenty of such sources. There were thirty incubator bassinets equipped with humidifiers drawing on water reservoirs, and there were fourteen sinks — one in each of the ten baby rooms, three in the central nursing station, and one in the gown room. And then there were the usual jugs of sterile water for washing the babies' eyes and for other medicative purposes. Dr. Gezon arranged for water samples from every possible source. That included two samples from each sink — one from the drain and one from the aerator on the faucet. The screens that diffuse the water in an aerator can provide a water bug like Pesudomonas with an excellent breeding place. For good measure, he took a swab of the respirator used in the ward. Also, Dr. Rycheck said, Dr. Gezon arranged for throat and stool samples from the two residents and from all the nurses working in the premature nursery. And he had called another meeting for Monday morning. The laboratory findings would be ready for evaluation by then.

"I made the Monday meeting. The laboratory reports were presented, and then we tried to decide what they meant. The human studies made pretty plain reading. There were two sets — the nurses and residents, and the twenty-eight seemingly well babies in the nursery. The laboratory eliminated the nurses and residents as possible carriers. Their cultured specimens were all negative for Pseudomonas. The reports on the babies confirmed what I think most of us had already suspected. This was a real epidemic. Twenty-two of the babies were negative for Pseudomonas, but six were positive. They weren't clinically sick. They didn't show any symptoms. They were, however, infected with Ps. aeruginosa. Why they weren't sick is hard to say. There were several possible explanations. The best one was that their exposure was relatively slight and their natural defenses were strong — they hadn't been weakened by antibiotics. The results of the environmental studies were very interesting. But they were also rather confusing. They showed five sink drains and three of the bassinet reservoirs to be contaminated. Everything else was negative for Pseudomonas — the water jugs, the respirator, the faucet aerators, and the other drains and bassinets. The contaminated drains were in Room 207, Room 209, Room 227, an unoccupied room, and the gown room. The contaminated bassinets were in 224, 227, and 229. All the infected babies were associated with just two rooms. They were, or had been, in either Room 227 — the room where the first baby took sick — or Room 229, where he died and where the two other babies became sick. There was a contaminated sink in Room 227, but the sink in 229 was clean. There was a contaminated bassinet reservoir in each room, but only one of the bassinets was, or had been, occupied by an infected baby. There were no infected babies in two rooms — Room 209 and Room 207 — that had contaminated sinks, and none in Room 224, which had a contaminated bassinet. It was all very peculiar. We had a lot of contamination and we had a lot of infected babies, but there didn't seem to be any connection between the two. The only link we could think of was the nurses. The babies had no contact with each other. The bassinets were self-contained, and none of the babies shared any equipment or medication. The nurses might have carried the infection on their hands. They could do that without becoming infected themselves. Healthy adults don't succumb to Pseudomonas. But why did they carry it only to the babies in 227 and 229?

"The meeting ended on that unsatisfactory note. Dr. Gezon was as puzzled as the rest of us. But, of course, this puzzling point was only part of the investigation. We still had an epidemic to contain. We didn't understand the mechanics of its spread, but we did know what it was, and we thought we had enough information to bring it under control. We knew who was sick and we knew that the nursery was contaminated at eight specific sites. By Monday night, the nursery was as clean as Dr. Gezon and the nursery staff knew how to make it. All the sinks were scrubbed with sodium-hypochlorite disinfectant. The bassinet reservoirs were emptied and disinfected with an iodophor, and only those in use were refilled. As a further precaution, that water was to be changed every day. Certain nurses were assigned to take exclusive care of the infected babies. Also, in the hope of dislodging their infection, all the infected babies were placed on a five-day course of colistimethate given intramuscularly, and colistin sulphate by mouth. It wasn't necessary to isolate the infected babies. They were already isolated. And it was arranged that specimens be taken every day from all the babies in the nursery, and from all the sinks and bassinets and so on. That would give us a constant focus on the course of the epidemic.

"I didn't participate in the sanitation program. They didn't need me. I would have been an extra thumb. I went back to my office and back to the regular Health Department routine, but part of my mind was still out there at the nursery, and I got to thinking about something I'd read a few months before. It was a report in the *Lancet* about an outbreak of Pseudomonas in an English nursery that was traced to a catheter used to relieve throat congestion in the babies. The source of the trouble eluded detection for almost a year. What I particularly remembered about the report was a description of a new system of microbial identification. There are several different types of Ps. aeruginosa, and this report told how they could be differentiated by a laboratory procedure called pyocine typing. Pyocine typing makes use of the fact that certain strains of Pseudomonas will kill or inhibit the growth of other Pseudomonas strains, and it's a complicated procedure. Well, it occurred to me that pyocine typing might help to clarify our problem. It could at least tell us if all the sinks and all the bassinets and all the infected babies were infected with the same strain of Pseudomonas. I thought about it, and finally I called up Dr. Gezon. He saw the point at once. But, as I say, pyocine typing was then very new, and we didn't know where to turn for help. It could be that the system was being used only in England. We talked it over and decided that the best place to begin was at the Communicable Disease Center, in Atlanta. If anybody was doing pyocine typing in this country, the people there would certainly know. That was Monday evening. On Tuesday morning, I got on the phone to Atlanta and talked to one of my friends at CDC and asked him what he knew about something called pyocine typing. 'Pyocine typing?' he said. 'Why, Shulman is working on that right now. I'll switch you over to him.' Shulman was Dr. Jonas A. Shulman, and a fellow Epidemic Intelligence Service officer. He's now assistant professor of preventive medicine at Emory University. I described the case to him and asked him if he could help us out, and he was more than willing. He was eager. He wanted all the work he could get. So as soon as we finished talking I arranged for specimens of all our isolates to be air-mailed down to Atlanta. Pyocine typing takes about two days. Shulman might have something for us by Thursday.

"Before I left the hospital, I went around to the premature nursery. That *Lancet* paper was still on my mind. Not pyocine typing. What interested me now was the source of the outbreak it described — that contaminated catheter. I looked up one of the pediatric residents and asked him what went on in the delivery rooms. I was thinking about contaminated equipment that the babies might have shared. For example, did they use a regular aspirator? The resident said no. The aspirators they used were all disposable and were discarded after each use. What about the resuscitators? Did they have humidifying attachments? A humidifier would mean water, and a possible breeding place for Pseudomonas, Another no. The resuscitators used in the delivery rooms were simply bags and masks attached to an oxygen line from the wall. I asked a few more questions along those lines and got the same kind of answers, and gave up. This wasn't a case like the *Lancet* case. So I was back in the nursery again. But the more I thought about those contaminated sinks and bassinets the less convinced I was that they were the source of our trouble. I just couldn't see any plausible link between those particular sites and those nine particular babies. But if the answer wasn't a piece of contaminated equipment, what else could it be? A contaminated person? And then I got a thought — maybe a contaminated mother. It sounded only too possible. A contaminated mother could very easily transmit an infection to her baby in the course of its birth. Childbirth is not a very tidy process.

"The next question was: Which mother? I thought I could answer that. It had to be the mother of the second sick baby. Not the baby in whom the infection was first diagnosed. The significant case was the second Pseudomonas baby — the term baby who came into the nursery with pneumonia and then developed diarrhea. The first sick baby had been healthy until the day before his death. He had been healthy for over three weeks. So he was actually No. 2. It wasn't hard to reconstruct the possible course of events. The infection was introduced into the nursery by the term baby and then spread to the other babies by the nurses. Pseudomonas is a difficult organism. You can't wash it off your hands with a little soap and water, the way you can the staphylococcus bug. To get Pseudomonas off, you have to scrub and scrub and scrub. And it's also extremely resistant to most disinfectants. But what made the infected-mother theory really attractive was that it seemed to explain what the environmental theory left unexplained. It explained why the infected babies were concentrated in Room 227 and Room 229. Both of those rooms were intensive-care rooms, and there was very little traffic between them and the other rooms. However, it was just a theory. It was based on the supposition that the diarrheal baby's mother was a Pseudomonas carrier. So the next thing to do was find out. The first thing I found was that the baby had been discharged on Saturday, and that he and his mother were now at home. I got the address, and Dr. Taylor and the baby's pediatrician gave me the necessary permission. I went out to the house and introduced myself, and the mother was nice and cooperative, and I got the specimens I needed and took them back to the Health Department lab.

"She wasn't a carrier. The preliminary laboratory report on my specimens was negative for Pseudomonas. That was the following day — Wednesday afternoon. But by then it didn't matter. We had something much more interesting to think about. The way it happened was this. I was in the nursery that afternoon, and one of the residents came over and told me they had another infected baby. New babies had been coming along every day, of course, and this one was a term baby born on Monday and sent up to the premature nursery for special care.

33

He had had trouble breathing at birth, and had required extensive resuscitation in the delivery room. Well, a routine nasopharyngeal culture taken when he was admitted to the nursery had just been found to be positive for Pseudomonas. I looked at the resident and the resident looked at me. This was real news. That baby could not possibly have been infected in the nursery. The laboratory samples had been taken before he was even settled there. He could have been infected only in the delivery room. And there were just two possible sources of infection there. His mother was one, and the other was some piece of contaminated equipment. My guess was naturally the mother. I found out what room the new baby's mother was in, and made the necessary arrangements, and went up and took the standard nose, throat, and stool samples, and arranged for the hospital laboratory to culture them. When I got back to the nursery, Dr. Gezon was there talking to the resident, and I could tell from the look on his face that he had heard the news.

"The three of us went down to the delivery suite. We found the nurse in charge and told her what we were doing. She was terribly upset. It was most distressing to her to have us arrive in her domain on such a mission. But she was a good nurse and she cooperated perfectly. The room where the baby had been born was not in use, and she took us in and showed us around. There was a delivery table in the middle of the room, and a row of scrub sinks along the left-hand wall. On the opposite wall was a resuscitator of the type described to me the day before. It consisted of a rubber face mask and a rubber Emerson bag enclosed in a cellophane casing, and it looked very neat and clean. But something made me take it down for a closer look. There was a little dribble of water in the bottom of the Emerson bag. I showed it to Dr. Gezon, and he raised his eyebrows and passed it on to the resident. The resident took a sample of the water. There were five other rooms in the delivery suite, and luckily none of them were in use. We checked the resuscitator in every room, and every one was wet. The question was: How come? The nurse explained the delivery-suite cleaning procedure. There was one central wash sink, where all delivery-room equipment was washed. Everything was washed after every use, and then sterilized by steaming in an autoclave. Including the resuscitators? No — of course not. They were made of rubber, and rubber can't stand that kind of heat. The resuscitators were washed with a detergent, rinsed with tap water, and left on the drainboard to dry. It was possible, the nurse said, that they were sometimes returned to the delivery rooms before they were completely dry. We asked to see the wash sink. We were all beginning to feel sort of elated. I know I was. And when we saw the sink, that just about finished us. The faucet was equipped with an aerator — a standard five-screen water-bug heaven.

"It *was* a water-bug heaven. The laboratory cultured Pseudomonas from the swab samples we took from the aerator. It also cultured Pseudomonas from five of the six resuscitator samples. You can imagine how the delivery-suite nurses felt when those reports came down. They were crushed. Dr. Gezon was able to reassure them, though. He didn't consider them guilty of negligence. He considered them guilty of ignorance. They assumed, like almost everybody else, that city drinking water is safe. It is and it isn't. It's perfectly safe to drink, but it isn't absolutely pure. This is something that has only recently been recognized. There are water bugs in even the best city water. The concentrations are much too low in ordinary circumstances to cause any trouble, but a dangerous concentration can occur in any situation — like that provided by an aerator — that enables the bugs to accumulate and breed. An aerator is a handy device, but you'd probably be better off letting the water splash. It's certainly a device that a hospital can do without.

"The laboratory gave us three reports in all. The third was on the mother of the new baby. They found her negative for Pseudomonas, and that was welcome news. A positive culture from her would have been an awkward complication. Because everything else was very satisfactory. The contaminated resuscitators seemed to explain the concentration of infected babies in Room 227 and Room 229. Seven of the ten infected babies — including the diarrheal baby and the two that died — had received at least some resuscitation in the delivery room, and it was reasonable to suppose that the three others had got their infection from the resuscitated babies by way of the nurses. There's plenty of evidence for that in the literature. I remember one report that showed that nurses' hands were contaminated simply by changing the bedding of an infected patient. It was Dr. Shulman, however, who finally pinned it down. His pyocine typing confirmed the circumstantial evidence at every point. Shulman did two groups of studies for us — one on the original material I sent him, and then another on the new infected baby and the delivery-suite material. The results of his studies were doubly instructive. They identified the delivery-room resuscitators as the source of the epidemic, and they eliminated the contaminated sinks and bassinets in the nursery. The different pyocine types of Pseudomonas aeruginosa are indicated by numbers. The Pseudomonas strain cultured from the delivery-suite aerator was identified as Pyocine Type 4-6-8. So were the isolates from the resuscitator bags. And so were those of all of the infected babies. Type 4-6-8 was also recovered from two pieces of equipment in the nursery, but I think we can safely assume that they had been contaminated indirectly from the same delivery-room source. They were a bassinet used by an infected baby and the sink in Room 227. The other contaminations in the nursery were a wild variety of types — 6, 4-6, 6-8, 1-2-3-4-6-7-8, and 1-3-4-6-7-8. And where they came from wasn't much of a mystery. There was only one possible explanation. They came out of the water faucets, too."

That was the end of the formal investigation. It wasn't, however, the end of the trouble. The pockets of contamination in the sinks and elsewhere in the nursery and in the delivery suite were eliminated (and a system of ethylene-oxide sterilization set up for all resuscitation equipment), but the epidemic continued. In spite of the most sophisticated treatment (first with colistimethate and colistin sulphate, and then with colistin in combination with polymyxin B), the infected babies remained infected. Moreover, in the course of the next few weeks twelve new infections were discovered in the nursery. In two of the new victims, the infection developed into serious clinical illness. It was not until the middle of September, when the remaining infected babies were moved to an isolated ward in another part of the hospital, that the epidemic was finally brought under control.

Hospital infections of any kind are seldom easily cured. Pseudomonas aeruginosa is only somewhat more stubborn than such other institutional pathogens as Staphylococcus aureus and the many Salmonellae. These confined and yet all but

37

unextinguishable conflagrations are, in fact, the despair of modern medicine. They are also, as it happens, one of its own creations. The sullen phenomenon of hospital infection is a product equally of medical progress and of medical presumption. It has its roots in the chemotherapeutic revolution that began with the development of the sulfonamides during the middle nineteen-thirties, and in the elaboration of new life-saving and life-sustaining techniques (open-heart surgery, catheterization, intravenous feeding) that the new antibacterial drugs made possible, and it came into being with the failure of these drugs (largely through the development of resistance in once susceptible germs) to realize their original millennial promise. Its continuation reflects a drug-inspired persuasion that prevention is no longer superior to cure. "In the midst of the development of modern antibacterial agents, infection has flourished with a vigor that rivals the days of Semmelweis," Dr. Sol Haberman, director of the microbiology laboratories at Baylor University Medical Center, noted. "It would appear that the long sad history of disease transmission by attendants to the sick has been forgotten again."

# Shiver and Burn

It began with a touch of malaise. Mrs. Walter Wells (as I'll call her), the eighteen-year-old daughter of a recently retired Army sergeant, and the recent bride of a vacuum-cleaner salesman, woke up that morning — Saturday morning, May 22, 1965 — at her home in Cataula, Georgia, a village some ten miles north of Columbus, feeling tired and achy and listless. Her husband was sympathetic and encouraging. He said it was nothing to worry about. She had probably been working too hard. That, she knew, was true enough. She *had* been working hard. She and her husband had only just moved to Cataula. Her father, a widower, had been stationed at Fort Benning, about five miles south of Columbus, and until April 15, when he retired from the service and moved to Florida, they had shared his quarters there. The move and the job of


39

getting resettled had been exhausting work. Her husband was right; she was probably a little run-down, and she would take it easy for a while. She did, but her indisposition persisted. She felt no better the following day, or on Monday, or Tuesday, or Wednesday. On Thursday, she began to feel worse. She felt cold, and then flushed and hot. She took her temperature; it was 101 degrees. An hour later, it had risen to almost 102. Then it began to fall, and by evening it was back to normal. It was normal all the next day. Even the dragging malaise seemed to have lifted at last. For the first time in a week, she felt almost well. But the day after that — on Saturday, May 29 — her temperature rose again. When her husband came in from a round of afternoon calls, it had climbed past 103. It was also well beyond any easy explanation. He went to the telephone and called the doctor.

The doctor whom Wells called was a general practitioner in Columbus whose name, I'll say, is John Henry Page. As it happened, however, Dr. Page was out of town that day, and the call was taken by an associate in the emergency room at St. Francis Hospital in Columbus. The nature of Mrs. Wells's illness, as her husband described it, was not at all clear to the doctor, but high fever is always decisive, and he told Wells to bring her right in. She arrived with a temperature of just under 103. The only other physical abnormality that a preliminary examination showed was some tenderness over the lower abdomen. That, together with high fever, suggested the possibility of an infection in that area. So did her history. The doctor gathered from Mrs. Wells that some months before — in July 1964 — she had been treated at the Martin Army Hospital, at Fort Benning, for a urinary-tract infection of some kind. This, it seemed quite possible, might be a recurrence of that.

Dr. Page took over the case on Sunday morning. He found Mrs. Wells sitting up comfortably and looking far from seriously ill. She said she felt pretty good, and her temperature was down to normal. The absence of fever was an acceptable surprise. A glance at the record showed him that she had been treated with tetracycline at the time of admission, and tetracycline has the power to promptly lower fever (by destroying its microbial cause). An examination of her lower abdomen was additionally corroborative: it was still tender — exquisitely tender. Dr. Page saw no reason to dispute his associate's definition of her trouble. The signs and symptoms were all generally consistent with a urinary-tract infection. On Monday, however, her familiar discomforts returned. She felt chilly and full of fugitive aches and pains, and her temperature began to climb. It climbed to 103. But it was back to normal on Tuesday, and so was Mrs. Wells. Then, on Wednesday, her temperature rose again. It continued to fluctuate like that. It was up one day and down the next, and when it was down she felt fully recovered. She felt so well that she wanted to get up and go home. Dr. Page sat down in perplexity and reviewed the clinical and laboratory records of the case. There was nothing in either to explain its peculiar progress. The next time she asked to be discharged, he shrugged and made the necessary arrangements. It was not an unreasonable decision. A week of hospital care and treatment had achieved no apparent results. That was one reason. Another was that Mrs. Wells could not afford an indefinite hospital stay. She had no kind of hospitalization insurance. Before she departed, however, Dr.

Page stopped by with a word or two of advice. He hoped she was on the road to recovery, but, in his opinion, she hadn't reached it yet. He wanted her to rest as much as possible, and he wanted her to keep a close watch on her temperature. If she had another attack of fever, he wanted to know at once.

Mrs. Wells was discharged from St. Francis Hospital on Wednesday, June 9. Three days later, on Saturday afternoon, she telephoned Dr. Page at his office. She reminded him that he had asked her to call if her fever came back. Well, it had. To tell the truth, she had felt a little feverish on Thursday, but — Anyway, this was different. She had just taken her temperature, and it was almost 103. Dr. Page heard her with more sympathy than surprise. He had half expected such a call. He gave a reassuring grunt, and told her not to worry. Nevertheless, he added, it seemed inadvisable for her to stay on at home. Didn't she agree? Very well. He wanted her back in the hospital that evening — in the Columbus Medical Center hospital this time. Mrs. Wells was admitted there at about six o'clock. Her temperature had dropped somewhat by then. The hospital reading was 100.8. The only other physical abnormality noted at the admission examination was continued abdominal tenderness. There was thus, as far as Dr. Page could see, no reason to revise his earlier diagnosis. Mrs. Wells still appeared to be the victim of a urinary-tract infection. He did, however, choose to revise his therapeutic attack. Instead of tetracycline, he prescribed a course of sulfisoxazole and chloramphenicol. They seemed, temporarily, effective. Mrs. Wells felt pretty well on Sunday, and her temperature was normal all day. But the following day, as so often before, the chills and fever and aches and pains returned. And the day after that, as equally often before, the symptoms all vanished. The results of the usual laboratory tests were also consistently uninstructive. Mrs. Wells's white-blood-cell count was 9500 — a trifle high, but normal. Her hemoglobin levels were 10.2 and 9.5 grams percent — a trifle low, and indicative of some anemia. Her urine contained a few white blood cells, but not enough to be of any pathological significance. Toward the end of the week, another round of standard tests was made. With one exception, the immediate results were exactly as before. The exception was an insignificant decline in Mrs. Wells's white-blood-cell count.

That was on Friday, June 18. The next afternoon, Dr. Page received at his office a call from the Medical Center. His caller was the hospital pathologist. He was calling, he said, to make an addition to the laboratory report on Mrs. Wells. One of the laboratory technicians had been inspired to take a closer microscopic look at a sample of her blood. The pathologist cleared his throat.

"You know what that girl's got?" he said.

"I don't guess I do," Dr. Page said. "What?"

"She's got malaria."

"*Malaria?*"

"Malaria."

"No kidding," Dr. Page said. "Well, golly Pete."

"I'm sending a blood sample down to Fort Benning for a confirmatory study," the pathologist said, "but there's no doubt about it. It's malaria. I looked at the smear myself."

"You know something?" Dr. Page said. "I'll bet my granddaddy is squirming in his grave. My daddy, too, for that matter. They wouldn't know what to make of me. I mean, they both would have had her diagnosed by at least the second day. But I've never seen a case of malaria before."

Malaria (or ague, or marsh fever, or jungle fever, or Roman fever, or Cameroon fever, or Corsican fever, or intermittent fever, or paludism) is probably the greatest of the great pestilential fevers. It is certain that no other infectious disease has caused so much misery to so many millions of people for so many thousands of years. It is equally certain that none has had so great an impact on the course of human history. Malaria has changed the direction of history on innumerable occasions. It was largely responsible for the periodic decline of civilization in ancient Mesopotamia, and for the physical, intellectual, and moral debilitation that toppled Attic Greece and Imperial Rome. It was malaria that caused the death of Alexander the Great at thirty-three, at the apex of his conquest of Asia. Endemic malaria held back for many years the construction of the Panama Canal, and because it finally yielded to American rather than to French control, it made possible the precocious preeminence of the United States in Central American affairs. And it was chiefly because of malaria that Black Africa is still predominantly black. It made West and Central Africa the celebrated "white man's grave" of mid-Victorian lore.

The cause of malaria is a tiny protozoan microbe of the genus *Plasmodium*. Four species of this influential parasite find the human body a satisfactory habitat. They are *Plasmodium vivax*, *Plasmodium falciparum*, *Plasmodium malariae*, and *Plasmodium ovale*. The human body is not, however, their only dwelling place. They require for the full development of their parasitical potentialities a certain period of residence in the body of one or another of the sixty or seventy members of the ubiquitous *Anopheles* genus of mosquitoes. That is where they manifest the sexual side of their nature. It is also where most biographers of *P. vivax* and its fellow-plasmodia choose

44

to open their inspection of the organism. The microbe reaches there in a droplet of blood drawn by a female anopheles (anopheline males are vegetarian) from some malarial man. The mating of male and female plasmodia occurs in the stomach of the mosquito, and at once. The ultimate progeny of this urgent, if haphazard, union are sporelike organisms called sporozoites. After two or three weeks, they gravitate by the thousand to stations in the salivary glands of the mosquito. From there, when next the mosquito feeds on human blood, they somehow insinuate themselves into the body of its victim. Once adrift in the bloodstream, these immigrant sporozoites move briskly with the circulation to a lodging in the functional cells of the liver. A leisurely period (six to twelve days) of growth and multiplication (by simple division) ensues. The fruits of this sojourn then burst from the ravaged cells and plunge into the bloodstream again. Some of these multitudes are recalled by chance or atavistic instinct to the liver, but most of them establish themselves in the red blood cells and settle down to another period of parasitic gourmandizing and asexual reproduction. This period, like the liver stage, ends with the disintegration of the victimized cells and the release of another generation of avid young plasmodia. It is the aim of each of these creatures to find and quickly penetrate another red blood cell and there repeat its reproductive cycle, but only a fraction succeed in doing so. About ninety percent of them are overwhelmed and destroyed by certain cells known as macrophages that the body summons into defensive action. Nevertheless, enough plasmodia survive this and subsequent macrophage attacks to insure an almost infinite continuation of their red-cell reproductive cycle. Three or four cycles, however, are usually sufficient to complete the evolution of the organism. The third or fourth cycle produces, in addition to the usual red-cell parasites, a number of sexually differentiated plasmodia. It is the chance ingestion of these fully evolved plasmodia by a feeding anopheles that perpetuates malaria.

Although all plasmodia are equally bound to this stylized mode of life, the different species follow it in somewhat different ways. Their differences in man are most pronounced in the red-cell reproductive stage. One point of difference is the age of the cell they choose to parasitize. *P. vivax* confines its insinuations to young and newly fabricated cells. So, it is believed, does *P. ovale*. *P. malariae*, on the other hand, is partial to cells that have reached maturity. Red blood cells of any age are acceptable to *P. falciparum*. Another difference in the species is their reproductive rate. *P. vivax* produces an average of sixteen new organisms in each invaded cell, but the average for *P. ovale* and *P. malariae* is only eight, and *P. falciparum* produces variously from eight to twenty-four. A third difference is in the length of the reproductive cycle. It ranges from between thirty-six and forty-eight hours for *P. falciparum*, through forty-eight hours for *P. vivax* and *P. ovale*, to seventy-two hours for *P. malariae*. These differences, though unimposing, are not without significance. They have sufficient impact to shape four more or less distinctive varieties of malaria.

The immediate cause of the clinical symptoms of malaria appears to be an acute intoxication. It is precipitated by the explosive end of the red-cell reproductive cycle and the sudden flooding of the bloodstream with obnoxious foreign protein — swarms of new plasmodia and cellular flotsam. The paroxysm of chills and fever that classically marks an attack of malaria thus is probably a toxic reaction. This reaction continues until the body's macrophage defenses have checked the swarming plasmodia and a kind of filtering service situated in the spleen (an enlarged and tender spleen is one of the clinical indications of malaria) has gathered up the debris. The nature of the reaction is largely determined by the nature of the infecting organism. *P. falciparum* has the most ferocious nature of its kind, and it induces by far the severest form of malaria — a form that is frequently fatal. One reason for this is the ready acceptance by the organism of any red cell, its high fertility, and the speed of its reproductive cycle. Another, and more important, reason is that in *P. falciparum* infections the red blood cells are so seriously affected that they tend to adhere to the walls of the capillaries and build a strangling occlusion. *P. vivax* and *P. ovale*, whose generative eruptions occur every other day, and *P. malariae*, with a cycle that produces in its victims a paroxysm only every third day, lack this sinister agglutinative power (as well, perhaps, as other, still incompletely fathomed powers), and the malarias they produce are relatively (though only in comparison with falciparum malaria) less severe. They, too, can be fatal, they are almost always prostrating, and they tend (if untreated) to hang on for months, and sometimes even years.

The regular recurrence of chills and fever at intervals of a day or two or three is classically suggestive of malaria. With the possible exception of the afternoon rise in temperature that traditionally characterizes tuberculosis, a predictably intermittent fever occurs in no other disease. It sets malaria distinctly apart from fevers of other origin. The uniqueness of malaria in this respect made possible its early recognition as an entity. It seems to have been recognized as such at least as early as the fifth pre-Christian century. The Book of Leviticus, which was written at about that time, contains a probable allusion to malaria in one of the several instances on record there of the Lord's exceptional truculence: "I will even appoint over you terror, consumption, and the burning ague." It is certain that malaria was specifically known to Hippocrates. In *Epidemics I*, his masterwork, he clearly distinguishes between continuous and intermittent fevers. He then defines the intermittent fevers as quotidian (daily), tertian (every third day), quartan (every fourth day), and semi-tertian. A semitertian fever is one that recurs about every thirty-six hours, like that of falciparum malaria. "The least dangerous of all," he reports, "and the mildest and most protracted, is the quartan. . . . What is called the semi-tertian . . . is the most fatal." The first-century Roman encyclopedist Aulus Cornelius Celsus saw malaria even more plainly. "Of fevers," he wrote in *De Medicina*, a medical compendium, "one is quotidian, another tertian, a third quartan. . . . Quartan fevers have the simpler characteristics. Nearly always they begin with shivering, then heat breaks out, and, the fever having ended, there are two days free; thus on the fourth day it recurs. But of tertian fevers there are two classes. The one, beginning and desisting in the same way as quartan, has merely this distinction, that it affords one day free, and recurs on the third day. The other is far more pernicious. . . . Out of forty-eight hours, about thirty-six . . . are occupied by the paroxysm." An association between malarial fevers and swamps and marshes was also observed very early. One of the most precocious of these observers was a Roman scholar of the first pre-Christian century named Marcus Terentius Varro. In discussing the proper site for a farmhouse, Varro warns, "Note also if there be any swampy ground . . . because certain minute animals, invisible to the eye, breed there . . . and cause diseases that are difficult to be rid of. Said Fundanius: 'What shall I do to escape malaria, if I am left an estate of such a kind?' 'Why,' said Agrius . . . 'you must sell it for as [much] as you can get, or if you can't sell it, you must quit it.' " A century later, Lucius Junius Moderatus Columella, a Hispano-Roman writer on agricultural subjects, came independently to the same supposition. "Nor indeed must there be a marsh near the building," he declared, "for [a marsh] always throws up noxious and poisonous steams during the heats." And, he perspicaciously added, it "breeds animals with mischievous stings which fly upon us in exceeding thick swarms . . . whereby hidden diseases are often contracted."

The Roman implication of "certain minute animals" and "animals with mischievous stings" in the spread of malaria vanished from the European mind with the fall of the Roman Empire. It was lost, along with most of the rational arts and sciences of Greco-Roman culture, in the credulities of medieval Christianity until almost modern times. All that survived of the observations of Varro and Columella (and many others of their inquisitive kind and time) was a vague distrust of marshy places as a source of malarial steams. The name "malaria," as it happens, derives from this miasmal theory. It developed from the Italian *mala* (bad) and *aria* (air), and was introduced into English by Horace Walpole in a letter to a friend (". . . a horrid thing called mal'aria, that comes to Rome every summer and kills one") in 1740. The traditional French designation of the disease, *fièvre paludéenne* (or marsh fever), is equally miasmal. There was a time, however, in the deeps of the Middle Ages, when even the miasmal explanation of malaria slipped from common knowledge. Malaria then was taken to be a form of demonic possession. The sudden chill, the blaze of fever, the burst of sweating, and then the almost instantaneous recovery suggested to innocent imaginations the malicious coming and going of a fiend, and charms were composed to hasten his departure. One — to be chanted up the chimney — ran:

> Tremble and go!
> First day, shiver and burn,
> Tremble and quake!
> Second day, shiver and learn,
> Tremble and die!
> Third day, never return.

Almost two thousand years went by before the possibility of a connection between mosquitoes and malaria was once more glimpsed and recorded. Giovanni Maria Lancisi, an early-eighteenth-century Italian epidemiologist and physician to three popes (Innocent XI, Clement XI, and Innocent XII), is usually celebrated as Columella's most immediate successor. In 1717, in an examination of the miasma theory entitled "De Noxiis Paludum Effluvis," Lancisi confidently traced the source of malaria to marshes and other stagnant waters, and then proposed that the mosquitoes so abundant there might be the agents of its dissemination. He also described the nature of their role. Mosquitoes "do not cause death by the bite or the wound," he declared, "but infuse by the bite or wound a poisonous fluid into our vessels." Lancisi's recovery of the ancient Roman comprehension of malaria was widely read and warmly proclaimed, but it failed to excite emulation. "De Noxiis Paludum Effluvis" at once became the standard word on the subject, and it remained about the only one for well over a hundred years. Then, in 1854, a West Indian physician of French extraction named Louis Daniel Beauperthuy perceived a larger measure of the truth. "The absence of mosquitoes during cold weather explains the disappearance of malaria," he wrote at the end of a study in Venezuela. "Intermittent fever is a serious disease spread by and due to the prevalence of mosquitoes. . . . [It owes its] toxicity to an animal or vegeto-animal virus, the introduction of which into the human system occurs by inoculation. The poisonous agent, after an incubation period, sets up . . . a true decomposition of the blood." Beauperthuy (if he meant what he seems to say) was one of the brilliant guessers of prescientific medicine. He died, in 1871, on the eve of the establishment of the germ theory of disease causation, and the triumphant riddling of malaria in the closing years of the nineteenth century was — and could only have been — a product of modern medical science. It was also, as is usual in modern science, the work of many men in many parts of the world. They included Rudolf Leuckart, a pioneer German parasitologist (who showed, by way of a worm parasite of fish that also lived in a species of flea, that an insect could serve as intermediate host to an animal parasite); Patrick Manson, a Scottish physician working in China who showed, through studies of a nematode infestation (called filariasis, that a mosquito could extract a parasite from the blood of a man and then satisfactorily serve it as a host); the American pathologists Theobald Smith and F. L. Kilborne (who showed, in a series of experiments with cattle, that insects can transmit disease from one animal to another); Charles Louis Alphonse Laveran, a French Army physician working in Algeria (who showed the presence of protozoa of the genus *Plasmodium* in the red blood cells of a malaria patient); Camillo Golgi, an Italian histologist (who showed that the malaria paroxysm coincides with the release of plasmodia from the parasitized red cells); and Ronald Ross, a Scottish surgeon in the Indian Medical Service. It was Ross's discovery of plasmodia in the stomachs and, a year or two later, plasmodia spores in the salivary glands of anopheles mosquitoes that had fed on malaria patients which completed the general elucidation of the disease. The first of these climactic discoveries was made on August 21, 1897, and on the evening of that day he cautiously announced the fact in a letter to his wife, in England: "I have seen something very promising indeed in my new mosquitoes." He then turned to his journal and, in the privacy of its pages, opened his heart in a poem:

> This day designing God
> Hath put into my hand
> A wondrous thing. At His command
> I have found thy secret deeds
> Oh million-murdering Death.
>
> I know this little thing
> A million men will save —
> Oh death where is thy sting?
> Thy victory oh grave?

Ross was, providentially, a better prophet than poet. His divinely directed discovery, by finally and firmly fixing attention on the anopheles mosquito as the vector in malaria, has unquestionably saved many millions of men. It is probable, however, that many millions more owe their salvation to modern adaptations of two weapons that have been at hand for centuries. One of these came into being as a natural corollary of the miasma theory. This, in its earliest effective form, was the draining of marshes. The other, of course, is quinine. Quinine is a complicated alkaloidal compound ($C_{20}H_{24}N_2O_2$) that was originally derived from the bark of the cinchona tree, a South American evergreen indigenous to Peru. The first malarial European to experience the power of an infusion of cinchona bark to block or terminate a paroxysm of chills and fever was a Jesuit missionary named Juan Lopez. That was in 1600. The healing draught was given to Lopez by a friendly Peruvian Indian, but how the Indian knew of its curative powers is uncertain. Malaria is not native to the Western Hemisphere. It entered the New World in the blood of the Spanish conquerors of Mexico and Peru in the sixteenth century, and it seems unlikely that the remnant Incas could have become sufficiently familiar with the new disease by the time Lopez was felled to know its specific vulnerability to cinchona bark. The probability is that his benefactor merely knew the bark to possess (as it does) a cooling touch in fever. Cinchona bark was introduced into Europe by Alonso Messias Venegas, another Jesuit missionary, in 1632. Its mastery of malaria was quickly confirmed and ardently endorsed by a succession of ailing Jesuits, including Cardinal Juan di Lugo, the illustrious confidant of Innocent X. Outside the Society of Jesus, however, the bark was for a time rather differently received. Its Jesuitic genesis rendered it repellent to many seventeenth-century Protestants. Oliver Cromwell was an outstanding member of that fiercely sectarian company. He died, in 1658, of malaria, after refusing a proffered decoction of what he (and others of his kind) called Jesuits' bark. Cinchona bark, or Jesuits' bark, or (as it most generally came to be known) Peruvian bark, was also rejected on principle by much of seventeenth-century medicine. Orthodox medicine found its action not in harmony with the rationale of therapeutics then in vogue. This rationale was venerably rooted in the humoral theory of pathology, which held that disease resulted from an imbalance of the body's constituent fluids (originally

53

blood, phlegm, yellow bile, and black bile), and it conceived the function of a drug to be the restoration of balance by seeking out and neutralizing harmful substances and then eliminating them from the body by means of violent purgation — by inducing vomiting, sweating, salivation, urination, hemorrhage. The conventional treatment of malaria included a powerful calomel purge. Humoral pathology dominated medicine until the establishment by Rudolf Virchow and others of cellular pathology around the middle of the nineteenth century, but the eventual acceptance of Peruvian bark — along with such other non-purgative specifics as colchicum (for gout) and digitalis — served to hasten its end. Peruvian bark was itself supplanted in the early nineteenth century. In 1820, the French pharmacologists Pierre Joseph Pelletier and Joseph Bienaimé Caventou discovered in quinine, an isolated essence of the bark, a more potent and more potable remedy for malaria, and within three years it was widely manufactured and almost everywhere available. The ingenuities of modern chemistry have since produced a synthetic quinine and a multitude of other remedies. Among the most esteemed of these are chloroquine, amodiaquine, and primaquine. Chloroquine and amodiaquine are substitutes for quinine. Like quinine, they are able, by destroying plasmodia of all species in the red-cell reproductive stage, to swiftly cure an acute attack of malaria, but they have no effect on the reservoir of plasmodia sequestered in the liver. The powers of primaquine are precisely supplemental to those of the quininelike drugs. Primaquine is lethal to the liver-dwelling plasmodia, and it can also kill or sterilize the sexually mature products of the red-cell stage — the organisms whose ingestion by an anopheles mosquito perpetuates the disease. Eight to ten days of quinine (or three days of one of its companion drugs) followed by fourteen days of primaquine will usually effect a radical, or total, cure.

Sanitary engineering, insecticides such as DDT, and the several antimalarial drugs have saved many millions of lives around the world, but they have also done more than that. They have made the lives of many more millions bearable. The menace of malaria is not so much its frequent lethality as its far more common capacity for taking the life out of living. No disease is more dulling, more depressing, more debilitating than chronic malaria. It was malaria in its chronic form that crushed the spirit of Attic Greece and wasted the strength of Rome, and practically every habitable part of the world (with the unexplained exception of New Zealand and most of the islands of Oceania) has at some time felt its enervating touch. "An intensely malarial locality cannot thrive," Ronald Ross wrote in a monograph in 1907. "The children are wretched, the adults frequently racked with fever, and the whole place shunned whenever possible by the neighbors. The landowner, the traveller, the innkeeper, the trader fly from it. Gradually it becomes depopulated and untilled, the home only of the most wretched peasants." J. A. Sinton, another British malariologist with wide experience in India, has offered a more comprehensive definition. "There is no aspect of life in [a malarial] country which is not affected, either directly or indirectly, by this disease," he noted, in 1936. "It constitutes one of the most important causes of economic misfortune, engendering poverty, diminishing the quantity and the quality of the food supply, lowering the physical and intellectual standard of the nation, and hampering increased prosperity and economic progress in every way." An anonymous traveler on the Mississippi River in the eighteen-thirties (presented by Erwin H. Ackerknecht in *Malaria in the Upper Mississippi Valley: 1760–1900*) has durably described the look of chronic malaria. "As we drew near Burlington, in front of a little hut on the riverbank sat a girl and a lad — most pitiable-looking objects, uncared-for, hollow-eyed, sallow-faced," this memoirist wrote. "They had crawled out into the warm sun with chattering teeth to see the boat pass. To Mother's inquiries the captain said: 'If you've never seen that kind of sickness I reckon you must be Yankee. That's the ague. I'm feared you will see plenty of it if you stay long in these parts. They call it here the swamp devil, and it will take the roses out of the cheeks of these plump little ones of yours mighty quick. Cure it? No, Madam. No cure for it: have to wear it out.'" Children are particularly enfeebled by chronic malaria. "Chronic malaria in children retards normal growth," Paul F. Russell and his collaborators point out in *Practical Malariology*, the standard modern work in the field. "Such children are often listless, with sallow, puffy faces, thin, flaccid muscles, protuberant abdomen, and pale mucous membranes. Liver and spleen are enlarged, the latter sometimes enormously. Anorexia [loss of appetite], dyspepsia, and flatulence are common. Fever is recurrent. If untreated, the condition . . . may result in early death."

Malaria reached its broadest sweep around the middle of the nineteenth century. It was all but universal. It was endemic almost everywhere in Asia, Africa, and Latin America; in Mediterranean Europe (the fever of which Byron died at Missolonghi in 1824 was malaria) and in much of Russia, Germany, Holland, and England (malaria accounted for five or six of every hundred patients treated at St. Thomas's Hospital in London between 1850 and 1860); and in most of the United

States. Its grip then somewhat loosened, and by the end of the nineteenth century the disease had largely disappeared from northern Europe, and in the United States it was still endemic only in the South. This salubrious, if circumscribed, decline has been variously explained, but most authorities attribute it to such fruits of industrialization as fewer swamps, better drains, less porous houses, more plentiful quinine, an intenser cultivation of land, and the displacement of riverboats by trains. In other, less dynamic parts of the world (including the American South), the spread of malaria was wholly unimpeded until shortly after the Second World War. As recently as 1940, some hundred and fifty thousand cases of malaria were reported in the United States, practically all of them in the South, and it is certain that there were many times that many cases not reported. Ten years later, in 1950, a more reliable method of reporting turned up a mere two thousand cases. There were fewer than two hundred in 1965. The therapeutic impact of growth and industrialization — and quinine and primaquine and DDT — has also been felt in other malarial countries. Since 1949, when the World Health Organization of the United Nations launched its continuing program of malaria eradication, the disease has been more or less uprooted in much of South America, in most of the Western Mediterranean world (including the once notoriously pestilential island of Sardinia), and even in parts of Pakistan and India. WHO has estimated that some three hundred fifty million cases of malaria — three and a half million of them fatal — occurred throughout the world (exclusive of China, North Vietnam, and North Korea) in 1955. In 1965, the total (for the same world) was around a hundred million cases, with about a million deaths.

57

Malaria thus appears to be going, and going pretty fast. Nevertheless, it is still very far from gone. "If we take as our standard of importance the greatest harm to the greatest number," Sir Macfarlane Burnet noted in "The Natural History of Infectious Disease," in 1953, "then there is no question that malaria is the most important of all infectious diseases." His appraisal remains unquestioned. "Malaria has a higher morbidity rate and is responsible for more deaths per year than any other transmissible disease," Martin D. Young, a leading American malariologist and a member of the expert panel on malaria of WHO, noted in a monograph in 1960. And in 1965 Marcolino G. Candau, director-general of WHO, declared, "From a world-wide point of view, communicable diseases must certainly be considered the No. 1 health problem, and among them malaria holds the most prominent place." Malaria still flourishes, as it always has, in all but Saharan Africa, in Central America, in the Middle East, in most of Southeast Asia, and on some of the islands of the southwest Pacific. The reasons for its prevalence there are chiefly ignorance and indifference. The causes of its lingering presence elsewhere in the world are more varied and more complicated and, it may turn out, more serious. They include — as many recent studies, among them the investigation that illuminated the case of Mrs. Walter Wells, have shown — the appearance of anopheles mosquitoes that are resistant to DDT and other insecticides, the appearance of plasmodia resistant to therapeutic (or tolerable) doses of all known anti-malarial drugs, the appearance of monkeys that can harbor malarial parasites to which man is also hospitable, and the fact that in many places from which endemic malaria has long since been banished the anopheles mosquito continues to live and breed.

The investigation into the case of Mrs. Walter Wells began on Tuesday, June 22. It was undertaken — at the invitation of the Georgia State Department of Health, and the medical authorities at Fort Benning — by two epidemiologists in the Epidemiology Branch of the Communicable Disease Center of the United States Public Health Service, in Atlanta. They were Robert L. Kaiser, chief of the Center's Parasitic Disease Unit, and James P. Luby, an Epidemic Intelligence Service officer assigned to Dr. Kaiser's office. The field work fell to Dr. Luby.

"That was only natural," Dr. Luby says. "This wasn't the first case of malaria down around Fort Benning that we had been asked to investigate. They'd had another civilian case — also a woman — down there the year before, in the summer of 1964. The investigation was headed by an EIS officer named Myron Shultz — he's up in New York now — but I was in on it. It wasn't a great success. We finally had to write it off as a cryptic case. In other words, we couldn't find the source of her infection. This time, I didn't ask for much — just somebody recently sick with an explicable case of malaria, and some anopheles) mosquitoes in the right place at the right time to carry it to Mrs. Wells. But at least I knew the way to Columbus and some of the medical people there and out at the base. I got the assignment on Monday afternoon, and I drove down the following morning. Columbus is a good three hours from Atlanta. I checked in at one of those day-or-night motels that line the highway between Columbus and Fort Benning, and had an early lunch. Then I went on to the base and had a talk with the chief of preventive medicine there. That was Major Taras Nowosiwsky, one of the people I knew from the 1964 investigation. He showed me the laboratory data on the case.

59

As expected, the base had confirmed the finding at the Columbus Medical Center. The only thing new was the type. Mrs. Wells's malaria was vivax malaria. Major Nowosiwsky then took me around to pay my respects to the commanding medical officer at the Martin Army Hospital, and I gave them a rough idea of what I planned to do. They promised me every possible assistance. The fact that Mrs. Wells was a former army dependent gave them a certain sense of responsibility. My next stop was the Muscogee County Health Department, in Columbus. Mary John Tiller, the deputy commissioner, was another of my old friends, and she made me feel right at home. I remember the greeting she gave me. 'Well,' she said, 'I was wondering when somebody from CDC was going to show up.' My purpose in seeing Dr. Tiller was to try to get some idea of the probable scope of the problem. She put my mind at rest on that. The local papers and the radio had given Mrs. Wells and her case all kinds of publicity, and she had been the subject of a medical grand rounds at the Medical Center — all of which, incidentally, gives you a pretty good idea of how times have changed in malaria — but nothing else had been brought to light. So the chances were good that Mrs. Wells was all I had to worry about. I decided it was time I had a talk with her.

"I found Mrs. Wells sitting up in bed and looking pretty good. They had started her on chloroquine as soon as the diagnosis was made, and she was now on primaquine. She was still a little weak, but her temperature had been normal since Sunday, and the worst was obviously over. She was very nice and helpful. We went over her history together. I couldn't really blame Dr. Page for missing the diagnosis. Nobody thinks of malaria around here anymore. But here in Georgia was where Mrs. Wells had contracted malaria. Her history settled that. She hadn't been in any of the malarial countries. The only time she had ever been abroad was a trip to Germany with her father in 1960. Since then, she hadn't even been out of the state. It was also certain that she had contracted malaria in the usual way — from the bite of an infected mosquito. It is possible, you know, to get malaria by way of a blood transfusion or through an injection of some kind. The literature is full of drug addicts with malaria. And you may remember all that excitement up in New York a few years ago when they found a blood donor with malaria. But Mrs. Wells had no recent injections or transfusions in her history. She had had some recent illnesses, though. The most recent was some menstrual trouble back in January, shortly after her marriage. In September, when she was still living at the base, she had an attack of strep throat. The most interesting illness was one that began on July 8. That was very interesting. Her symptoms included chills, fever, backache, weakness, and urinary frequency, and, the way she remembered it, the fever was intermittent. She consulted the outpatient department at the Martin Army Hospital on the second day, and, apparently on the basis of that urinary complaint, the examining physician made a tentative diagnosis of urinary-tract infection. She was treated with antibiotics, and in about ten days she was well. One of the things that made that illness interesting was, of course, the symptoms — chills and intermittent fever. They were compatible with a urinary-tract infection when taken by themselves, but not when the record showed a urinalysis negative for white blood cells. The other thing was the date of onset. July 8, 1964, struck a certain chord in my memory. It reminded me of that other case of malaria I'd been in on. I'll call her Mrs. Durham. Mrs. Durham's onset was July 10, 1964.

"That gave me something to think about that evening after dinner. A good coincidence is always worth thinking about. Epidemiology is practically the science of coincidence. It was very hard to believe that those two cases of malaria were unrelated. Mrs. Wells's history suggested very persuasively that this attack of malaria was not her first attack. The primary attack had occurred in July of 1964. This attack was a recurrence of that infection. The fact that she had recovered from the first attack without specific treatment didn't in the least embarrass that hypothesis. Untreated malaria recurs and recurs, but each attack is self-limited. After a certain length of time, the red-cell stage of the organism simply peters out. But onset wasn't the only coincidence. There was also the disease itself. Mrs. Wells had vivax malaria. So did Mrs. Durham. Another coincidence was proximity. Mrs. Durham was the wife of a second lieutenant, and they lived in Battle Park Homes, a duplex development at the base for junior officers. Mrs. Wells also lived at the base in 1964 — in a development on Baker Street for noncommissioned officers. Battle Park Homes and Baker Street were only about a mile apart. Or so I gathered from Mrs. Wells. And most of the country in between was rough, heavily wooded, and full of damp, brushy hollows. It sounded just right for mosquitoes.

"I spent the next day in Cataula. Most of it, anyway. I would much rather have been poking around at Fort Benning, but it doesn't pay to cut corners. Before I went any further, I had to make completely certain that there hadn't been any other cases of malaria in the neighborhood. Cases that hadn't been diagnosed, that is, or asymptomatic cases. Dr. Tiller had arranged for the county sanitarian to show me around. A stranger, especially a stranger from up North — my home town is Chicago

— needs someone to vouch for him in those little Georgia towns. We met, and he took me around to meet the local physicians. There were two of them, a husband and wife in practice together, but they had nothing to contribute — no cases of malaria, no unexplained illnesses with fever, nothing in the least suspicious. That was as expected. They were mainly a courtesy call. If they had known any news, they wouldn't have saved it for me. Then we started in on our own. We started with Mrs. Wells's husband, then we saw his parents, then we called on the neighbors. Our procedure was this. We asked about any episode of fever in the recent past. If we got an affirmative answer, we asked about the cause. If the cause was unknown or uncertain, we took a sample of blood for definitive analysis. We visited forty-four homes within a mile-and-a-half radius of Mrs. Wells's home and we checked out a total of two hundred and fourteen people, but we didn't find a thing. There was one old man who had a suspicious history, and we got some blood and sent it back to the CDC laboratory in Atlanta. They did a malaria smear and a fluorescent antibody test, but the results were negative. Well, that, of course, was a great relief. Anything else would have been an awkward complication. This simplified the problem. It didn't tell us when Mrs. Wells got malaria. It was still possible that her present attack was her first. But it did tell us where. She got it at the base.

"I didn't believe that this was her first attack. But, as I say, it was possible. The incubation period in vivax malaria — the interval between the mosquito bite and the onset of symptoms — is usually about two weeks. Mrs. Wells moved off the base around the middle of April, and she didn't get sick until the twenty-second of May — almost six weeks later. That would seem to eliminate a 1965 infection, but it didn't. The reason was, she had gone back to the base. She went back several times. Her father had retired to Fort Myers or some such place in Florida, but Mrs. Wells still had her Baker Street friends. So 1965 was still at least conceivable. The only way to settle it was another fever survey. I might mention, by the way, that we hadn't forgotten the father. Dr. Kaiser had arranged for someone to look him up for an interview. I talked to Dr. Kaiser on Wednesday night and told him what I had learned and what I thought and what I planned to do next, and he completely shared my views. Then he told me about the father. His history and his blood were both negative for malaria.

"I drove down to the base the next morning and saw Major Nowosiwsky again. I told him I wanted to make a fever survey in the Baker Street area, and he OK'd the plan and arranged for one of his men to take me around. Then I asked about mosquitoes. I assumed they were there, they had to be there. But I wanted to know. Major Nowosiwsky took me in to see the base entomologist. He was a colonel — Colonel Petrakis — and he got out his records on the subject. The mosquitoes were there. Routine trapping in season for pest-control analysis regularly turned up several varieties of mosquito, and they included an anopheline — *Anopheles quadrimaculatus. A. quadrimaculatus* is one of about a dozen native American anopheles, and in this part of the country it's the most common. It had been trapped in several different traps, but the traps that interested me were those set up at the intersection of Fort Benning Road and Arrowhead Road and Custer Road, in Battle Park Homes. Fort Benning Road is one of the main thoroughfares in the reservation. Arrowhead Road is the only road to Battle Park Homes, and it's one of two roads to Baker Street. The other road to Baker Street is Custer Road. Colonel Petrakis's records also noted that larvae of *A. quadrimaculatus* had been found in a creek directly across from the Baker Street houses. I thanked the Colonel and picked up my guide and drove out to Baker Street feeling a whole lot better. You can't have malaria without a vector. The Baker Street survey was another Cataula. I had two opening questions this time. One was about unexplained fever. The other was about foreign travel — visits to endemic-malaria areas within the past three years. We visited sixty-one homes and talked to two hundred seventy-one people, and we found nineteen people who had been in endemic areas and two cases of recent and unexplained fever, but we didn't find any malaria. And that took care of 1965. Mrs. Wells's malaria was a 1964 infection. There was no other reasonable possibility. There was also no good reason now to doubt that her case and Mrs. Durham's were linked.

"The nature of the link wasn't hard to visualize. It couldn't have been one of the neighbors. My Baker Street survey and one just like it that was done the year before in Battle Park Homes eliminated that possibility. A common hypodermic needle or a common blood donor was also out of the picture. So, of course, was a visit to some endemic country. That seemed to identify the index case as a visitor to the general neighborhood of Battle Park Homes and Baker Street. It didn't much matter just where. Colonel Petrakis had demonstrated that there were potential vectors all over the area. I went back to Major Nowosiwsky, and he got out the records on all the men from overseas who had come down with malaria at the base in the past twelve months or so. There were quite a number of them, but only four were cases of vivax malaria.

The others were mostly falciparum-malaria cases. Incidentally, that's the big malaria problem in Vietnam right now, and I gather it's quite a problem. They're seeing falciparum malaria out there that doesn't respond like the others. However . . . I was looking for vivax cases and found just four. Two captains and two sergeants. But worse than that, I knew them — all but one of them. I remembered both sergeants and one of the captains from the report on the Durham investigation, and the investigation had excluded them as possible sources of Mrs. Durham's infection. They were infectious — they had what we call parasitemia, they had the parasite in their blood — at the wrong time. I'll tell you what I mean. There are two incubation periods to be considered in malaria — one for the development of the parasite in the mosquito and another for the development of the parasite in the man. Both of these periods vary in length, but the mosquito period is the most variable. It varies with the temperature of the air. In vivax malaria in that part of Georgia, it ranges from a month or more in cool weather to a minimum of nine days in June and July. The minimum incubation period in man is eight days. The sum of those minimums is the minimum total incubation interval, or seventeen days. That's the shortest possible interval that could elapse between the infection of the mosquito and the onset of illness in Mrs. Durham and Mrs. Wells. So the man we were looking for should have had parasitemia in June, but no later than the twenty-fourth. Well, both the sergeants failed to satisfy that criterion, and for the same reason. Their onsets came too late. One was on June 28, and the other was on July 28. The captain was too early. His onset came on April 4. And the new case, the other captain, was even more hopeless. His onset date was March 21, 1965.

"I drove back to Atlanta that night. The next day was Saturday. I called Dr. Kaiser and told him the story. It looked as if we were up against another cryptic case. I know he was disappointed, but I felt worse than that. It made me uncomfortable, too, to think of that anonymous index case wandering around somewhere. He might very well be an asymptomatic carrier. I'd done my best, though. There was nothing I could think of left to do. I started in on my report on Monday morning. When I had my notes in order, I got out our general file on malaria. I wanted to take another look at the report on the Durham investigation. But I never got that far — not that morning. I came across something I'd never seen before. Or if I had, I didn't remember. It was a routine National Malaria Surveillance Report from the Third Army Medical Laboratory at Fort McPherson, Georgia. It was dated August 1964, and it reported cases of malaria diagnosed at Army installations in June of that year. I'd seen many such reports. The cases are identified by name, rank, and station, and there is always a short travel history. What made me stop and look at this report was a station — Fort Benning. I didn't even know I was looking until I saw it. It was cited in the travel history of a sergeant I'll call Sergeant Evans. Sergeant Evans was stationed at Fort Campbell, Kentucky, and his case had been diagnosed at the hospital there on June 27. He had arrived at Fort Campbell on June 24. Before that, he had been stationed at Fort Benning. He had been there from May 9 until June 23. Before that, he had been in South Korea.

"I picked up the phone and put in a call to Fort Campbell. It was practically automatic. And I was lucky. Sergeant Evans was still stationed there, and they finally found him and brought him to the phone. I told him who I was and what I wanted to know. His memory of his Fort Benning experience was vague. He lived there in barracks near the parachute-jump towers. That was a mile or two beyond the intersection of Fort Benning Road and Arrowhead Road and Custer Road. No, he didn't know Mrs. Durham or Mrs. Wells, and he had never been to Battle Park Homes or in the Baker Street development. Not that he remembered, anyway. His duties kept him mostly in the area near his barracks. But he had a car — a convertible — and he did get off the base a few times. And when he did, he naturally came and went by way of Fort Benning Road. How else? He supposed he had sometimes been stopped at the stoplight there at the Arrowhead Road and Custer Road intersection. Yes, he had been sick at Fort Benning. He'd had spells of chills and fever off and on during most of June. No, he hadn't reported for treatment — not until he got up to Fort Campbell. He kept hoping each remission was the end. One of his worst spells hit him one evening when he was off the base on a picnic. He remembered driving back to the barracks and shaking so hard he could barely drive. Yes, he usually drove with the top down. Or else why have a convertible? I laughed and agreed and thanked him for his help and cooperation, and hung up.

"I just sat there at my desk for a minute. I don't mind saying I felt pretty good. Then I got up and went in and told Dr. Kaiser what had happened."

# The Santa Claus
# Specimen

The second monthly meeting in 1966 of the Committee on Infection Control of the Massachusetts General Hospital was held at noon on February 23 in a private dining room in the George Robert White Building, the administrative center of the hospital complex. It was attended by thirteen members. Among them were physicians representing the several hospital services (medicine, surgery, pediatrics, orthopedics, neurology, urology), the chief bacteriologist, the chief of pharmacy, two executive nurses, and the assistant director of the hospital and secretary of the committee, Joseph W. Degen. The principal item of business was a report from Dr. David J. Lang, assistant pediatrician at the hospital and an instructor in pediatrics at Harvard Medical School. Mr. Degen's account of that portion of the meeting read: "Dr. Lang reported on the incidence of *Salmonella cubana* in the Burnham units. Six pediatric patients have been affected since October 1965. The prior incidence of one pediatric patient and six adults over the term from April to October had been thought not connected. However, in the absence of finding any specific source for the Burnham episode, and in the presence of certain possible connections via various paths (food, vitamins, persons) of the latest to the earlier cases, there is some possibility of connection. This particular outbreak in the Burnham units seems now to have stopped. No evidence of personnel-contact faults or any vast breaks in techniques as causes have been uncovered. There was a resultant advantage in the 'sharpening up' of procedures for proper care."

*Salmonella cubana* is one of some twelve hundred species of bacteria that comprise the genus Salmonella. These microbes (whose name commemorates the nineteenth-century American pathologist Daniel Elmer Salmon) produce an acute gastroenteritis known to clinical medicine as salmonellosis. Salmonellosis is almost as common a form of food poisoning as that caused by the ubiquitous staphylococci, and it generally runs a far less commonplace course. When its victims are very old or very young, or debilitated by some other disease, it is not infrequently fatal. Practically all animals (including rats, snakes, and insects) are hospitable to the salmonellae, but the microbe seldom produces a perceptible disease in any host but man. The usual cause of human salmonellosis is infected (and insufficiently cooked) beef, pork, lamb, duck, turkey, chicken, and, particularly, eggs. Other causes include food or drink contaminated by the excreta of infected animals and by tainted equipment. The different Salmonella species are distinguished by a serotyping technique perfected by the Danish bacteriologist F. Kauffmann in 1941, and they are identified (with one or two exceptions) by geographical names that indicate where they were first isolated. All of the many salmonellae are equally pathogenic, but some are more widely distributed in nature than others. The most widely distributed in the United States is *Salmonella typhimurium*; others that are frequently isolated here and elsewhere include *S. newport, S. montevideo, S. anatum, S. oranienburg, S. panama, S. dublin, S. sandiego, S. bareilly, S. tennessee, S. moscow, S. derby,* and *S. heidelberg. S. cubana* is not a member of that cosmopolitan company. It was first encountered in 1946 in Cuba, and its recorded appearances outside that country have been relatively rare. In 1964, the most recent year of accurate record, there were some twenty-five thousand cases of salmonellosis reported in the United States. Only sixty of these were attributed to *S. cubana.*

Dr. Lang's report on the *S. cubana* outbreak in the Burnham units was the ambiguous result of almost a month of intensive investigation. He had received the assignment at a special meeting of the Infection Control Committee on January 31. That meeting had been called to consider an urgent memorandum from the chief bacteriologist, Dr. Lawrence J. Kunz. His memorandum read: "(1) Stool of Gail H. on Burnham 6 has Salmonella-like organism which is not in Salmonella groups A-E: *S. cubana*? (2) Patient P. has organism similar to *S. cubana.* (3) Patient F. has *S. cubana* in stool." The identification of *S. cubana* in the first two patients, Dr. Kunz noted, was tentative but probable. There was no question about the third patient. The presence of *S. cubana* had been demonstrated at the leading laboratory of its kind in the East, the New York Salmonella Center, at Beth Israel Hospital, in Manhattan. Discussion of the memorandum brought out that all of these patients were children, and all had been in the hospital — in the Burnham wing of the Vincent Memorial Hospital and Burnham Memorial for Children — for at least a week before the samples were taken for laboratory analysis. None of them had shown any signs or symptoms of salmonellosis at the time of admission. Two of these children were girls, one seven weeks old and the other eight weeks, and the third was a two-month-old boy. It was added that the boy was no longer a patient. He had died, after a hospital stay of eight days, on January 28.

Dr. Lang says: "That was when we recognized the outbreak as an outbreak. Those three children in the Burnham building brought it into focus. They did for me, all right. The Burnham units are my bailiwick. The seven previous cases had been too sporadic to make any great impression. I went down from the committee meeting and looked up the charts of those earlier patients. They didn't seem to have anything in common but an uncommon variety of salmonellosis. There were five females and two males in the group, and they ranged in age from one to seventy years. They had been admitted to the hospital at very various times. One came in in March, two in May, three in September, and one in October. And they were scattered all over the hospital. They were in Vincent, in Burnham, in White, and in Baker Memorial — in four of our six clinical buildings. Also, according to the records, four of the seven had shown symptoms suggestive of salmonellosis at admission. That wasn't what they were admitted for — they all had different diseases — but the symptoms were there on the charts. And one of the others had given a positive stool sample on the second day of hospitalization. In other words, according to the evidence, five of those seven patients had come into the hospital already infected with *S. cubana*. It was just the reverse with the children. It was just as obvious that they had acquired their infections *after* their admission. Which meant that this new outbreak, whatever its source, had its origin somewhere within the walls of the M. G. H.

"I wasn't too concerned about the seven earlier cases. I was interested — everything connected with a serotype as uncommon as *S. cubana* is interesting — but they could wait. The immediate problem was the outbreak here in the Burnham building. Three cases of the same unusual thing at the same time in the same building suggested the possibility of a common source. It also suggested the rather alarming possibility of an explosive outbreak. Another possibility was that there might be other cases here that we didn't know about, and that was the question that had to be answered first. It's always helpful to know the scope of a problem. But not only that. It was entirely possible that the answer might say something useful about the source of the trouble. There were at the moment three units — three floors — involved. The girls were on Burnham Five and Burnham Six, and the little boy had been on Burnham Four. His floor had a certain significance. One reason was that he was the newest case. Another was that there had been two Burnham patients among the earlier cases, and both of them had been on Burnham Four. I was particularly interested in the little boy's room. I was thinking along the lines of baby-to-baby transmission, and his room seemed to be a good place for a comprehensive study. It was a room for six, and it had five children in it now. I ordered stool cultures of them all. Then, for a larger picture, I ordered cultures of all the Burnham nurses and all the Burnham food-handlers. A Salmonella culture takes about two days to develop. The growth, if any, can then be identified as a salmonella. In some laboratories, including ours, the group to which it belongs can also be determined then. Specific serotyping takes about a week. But we would know in a couple of days if the survey had turned up anything that could be *S. cubana* — anything, that is, in Group G, the *S. cubana* group. This was Monday. We would have at least a clue by Wednesday. Meanwhile, we would do what we could to keep the outbreak under control. I sat down with the chief resident and wrote a notice for posting on all the Burnham floors. Then I had a conference with the Burnham chief of nursing. I gave her my ideas, and she drew up a set of emergency regulations."

The notice read: "Recently there have occurred several cases of diarrhea and infection caused by *Salmonella cubana* on the Children's Service. Although this does not represent a major problem or threat at the moment, we are taking certain public-health steps that will prevent the infection from spreading. We have restricted admissions to emergencies or serious problems until we clarify the extent of the problem. We anticipate that by the end of the week we will have a clearer picture of what needs to be done."

The emergency regulations read:

MEMO
To: All head nurses and supervisors — Burnham Units
From: Miss Grady
The following recommendations (outlined by Dr. Lang) are to be effective throughout the Burnham Units until further notice:
A. Strict isolation technique shall be carried out on all patients having loose stools.
B. Protective precautions are to be carried out for ALL patients.
C. General Controls:
  1. Admissions limited to emergency cases.

2. Cleaning of entire floor by Building Services.

3. Stool cultures on all patients before discharge.

4. All nursing staff having symptoms of diarrhea to be sent off duty until report of stool culture obtained.

5. Two rooms in the X-ray Department have been designated for all children having examination.

6. All children leaving Unit for tests in other departments shall be gowned.

7. Personnel transporting all patients from Unit shall be gowned.

8. The services of the evening volunteers shall be suspended until further notice.

Dr. Lang says: "After that, there was nothing to do about the outbreak but wait for the reports on the stool cultures. I had time to think about those earlier cases again. If five of the seven had been infected outside the hospital, *S. cubana* must have been out and around the town. In that case, what about the other Boston hospitals? It might be interesting to hear what they had to say. I sat down and called them up — Peter Bent Brigham, Boston City, Children's, Beth Israel. I called them all. And they all said no. *S. cubana?* Good heavens, they never saw cubana. Nobody did. *Cubana* was a very rare bird. All of which left me a bit confused. It was strange enough that we should have all these cases of *S. cubana*, but it was even stranger that nobody else had any. It made me wonder about those five apparently outside cases. Were they actually outside cases? Or had they somehow become infected in the hospital, too? That was a tempting idea. It would simplify things considerably. And yet, of course, it wasn't acceptable. The evidence was all against it. But how could I explain those infections when there wasn't any *cubana* anywhere else in the city? The answer was that I couldn't, and I decided not to try. I decided that one outbreak was all I could hope to handle.

"The first reports on the stool cultures came along, as expected, on Wednesday. Two of the five children in the dead boy's room were positive for Group-G salmonella. And, as serotyping subsequently showed, their salmonella was *S. cubana*. Everybody else — the other children in the room, the nurses, the orderlies, the kitchen people — was negative. I began to get a little excited. I thought I could see the beginning of a pattern. Two of the earlier cases — and both of them definitely hospital-acquired infections — had been Burnham patients. [If we're talking about the Original Seven, only one was a pediatric case, we said.] So were the three January cases. And now we had two more. That made seven cases clustered in a single building. It was possible that the cluster was just a freak of coincidence. But there was also another possibility. The cluster could also mean that the source of the trouble was right here on my own service. Only it didn't. A few days later, on Monday, February 7, I got a call from Dr. Kunz. His laboratory had uncovered another positive salmonella in the Group-G category. The new infection was unquestionably hospital-acquired, and the patient was an adult. He was a man of seventy-two, and he was in the Bulfinch Building. So that was the end of the promising Burnham pattern. We were right back where we had started. The outbreak was hospital-wide. The new case also put an end to the emergency in the Burnham units. I mean, the emergency regulations now seemed needlessly strict, and Miss Grady, the chief of nursing, and I drew up a modified set."

The new regulations read:

1. The Burnham will reopen for all admissions on February 10, but crowding will be avoided absolutely.

2. Children with positive Salmonella cultures will be transferred to White 12 with pediatric nurse in situ.

3. Strict isolation technique will be maintained as before on all patients having loose stools.

4. Control of visitors will continue as before, and community recreation activities remain suspended. *All* patients will remain restricted to bed area. Maintain handwashing strictly.

5. Stool cultures on all patients before discharge.

6. Regulations persist with regard to personnel who have gastro-intestinal symptoms.

7. *All* bottles will be prepared by nursing personnel, bottles for older children included. Details of this preparation will be given to head nurses.

8. All other regulations (travel to X-ray, gowns on children without diarrhea, etc.) are no longer in effect.

Dr. Lang says: "A hospital-wide outbreak implies a source of infection common to all the hospital units. There has to be a link between the cases. There are various possibilities, including human carriers, but the usual one, of course, is food — either food already contaminated or food contaminated in the course of preparation. In other words, the kitchen. But that didn't look very possible here. The source could hardly be some already contaminated food or drink. That would mean an explosion — not just a handful of cases. And it could hardly be a contaminated kitchen. Each of the clinical buildings at the M. G. H. has its own kitchen. Then I learned something that I hadn't known before. It was true that each of the clinical buildings had its own kitchen, but there was also a special-diet kitchen here that served *all* the buildings. You can imagine how I reacted to that. A special-diet kitchen could be the perfect answer. All serious cases at one time or another get something in the way of special food, and all of our *cubana* cases were serious cases. I went along on the diet-kitchen inspection myself. We arranged for all the people there to be cultured, and then we went through the kitchen. We couldn't have been more thorough. We looked at all the food and all the equipment and checked over all the procedures. We found a few minor breaks in technique, but that was all. A day or two later, the culture reports came in — all negative. No sign of any kind of salmonella anywhere in the diet kitchen. So that was another disappointment, another dead-end lead. The next one came from Dr. Kunz."

Dr. Kunz says: "We were talking about possibilities. Possible vehicles other than food. Salmonella can be transmitted in some damned weird ways. I remember an outbreak back in 1955 that was traced to baby Easter chicks. And that made me think of the Santa Claus patient. That's an annual practical joke. To me, it's an annual nuisance, which is probably why I hadn't thought to mention it to Dr. Lang before. Anyway, there's a tradition here at Mass General that Santa Claus turns up every Christmas as a patient. He usually turns up on the Surgical Service. The way it works is this. Some nurses and house officers on the Service find an empty bed and assign it to Mr. S. Claus and make up a chart and all the rest. They do a complete job. They concoct some crazy kind of specimen and send it down in Santa's name for analysis. Sometimes the lab technician will look at the identification and see the name S. Claus, and that's the end of the joke. But sometimes she doesn't notice the name and puts the specimen through the regular procedure. Then the joke is on her. On all of us here in the lab. The Christmas of 1965 was a little different. The specimen purported to be a sample of urine. The technician — a girl named Harriet Provine — saw the name, but wasn't too busy at the moment and so, just for fun, she went ahead and processed it. That was on Friday, and Christmas was on Saturday. On Monday morning, the head technician checked the holiday-weekend cultures, and when she came to Mr. S. Claus, she almost went through the roof. It wasn't just the name. It was the culture itself. The Santa Claus culture had grown an organism — a Group-G salmonella.

"The head technician came in and told me what had happened, and then she and I went over and saw Harriet. The rest of the sample, of course, was gone. Harriet had thrown it away. We don't keep the stuff after it's been planted. However, we did know where it came from. I got on the phone to the floor and talked to a nurse who was in on the joke, and she told me how they had made the specimen. She said it consisted of water, an intravenous multivitamin preparation, a pinch of powdered carmine dye for coloring, and a throat swab from one of the patients on the floor. Carmine is a red, nonabsorbent dye that is used internally in medicine to time and measure bowel action. Well, the recipe sounded plausible. I asked the nurse to send me down another swab from the patient, and went to work making up another specimen of Santa Claus's urine. I didn't use the throat swab in my reconstruction. I wanted that cultured separately. When I finished my specimen, I took it over to Harriet to culture."

Miss Provine says: "But it wasn't the same thing. I told Dr. Kunz that this wasn't it at all. It was the wrong color. It was red. The Santa Claus specimen was yellow. It really looked like urine."

Dr. Kunz says: "I may have got the proportions wrong. But that wouldn't make any difference. The ingredients were the thing. I told Harriet to go ahead and culture it. She also cultured the throat swab. And they both were negative for any kind of salmonella. I hadn't expected anything from the throat swab. After all, it came from a surgical patient. But the original Santa Claus specimen — I couldn't understand it at all. It didn't make any sense. It was totally inexplicable."

Dr. Lang says: "It was interesting, though. I thought it was well worth looking into further. I went up to the floor and talked to some of the people involved. I didn't learn much of anything — except that apparently Miss Provine had been right about the color of the reconstructed specimen. The nurse that Dr. Kunz talked to must have got two hoax specimens confused. The jokers had also faked a blood sample for the chemical laboratory, and that was where they had used the carmine dye. The urine sample had got its color simply from the vitamin preparation. I checked with the chemical lab, and they remembered the blood sample, but they hadn't bothered to test it. They had recognized the joke and thrown the stuff away. It seemed to me that there were still two possibilities — two possible vehicles for the Santa Claus *cubana*. That's what his salmonella turned out to be. One possibility was the water, and the other was the vitamin preparation. I couldn't help but think of water. It had been less than a year since the big Riverside, California, epidemic. That was an epidemic of *Salmonella typhimurium* that caused around fifteen thousand cases of illness, and it was traced to contaminated water. Contaminated municipal water. I don't mean that I suspected Boston city water. My idea was that the water might have become contaminated at some point leading into the hospital. It wasn't a very serious idea. It was extremely far-fetched, and I wasn't in the least surprised when it almost immediately collapsed. As soon as I asked about the hospital's water supply, I found that every building had its own connection with the city main. The vitamin preparation seemed to be a little more promising. I got the idea from a paper by Dr. Kunz. The paper was published back in 1955, but I remembered it. It described culturing salmonella from yeast. Yeast is an unlikely vehicle for salmonella, but Dr. Kunz had shown that it could be one, and yeast is a source of vitamin B, and vitamin B was included in the intravenous multivitamin preparation. The fact that Dr. Kunz's reconstructed specimen had been negative for salmonella wasn't necessarily final. It didn't necessarily mean that the preparation was uncontaminated. It could simply mean that the concentration of salmonella was extremely low, and that there was none or not enough in the sample he took for his culture. I made certain of a high concentration. I put fifty vials of the stuff through a millipore filter and then planted the residue in a culture flask. If there was any salmonella there, that would surely show it up. But there wasn't any there. The yeast was just another blind alley. The culture was negative.

"That was around the middle of February. I had been plugging away for two or three weeks and I'd run down every discernible lead, and the result was absolutely nothing. It began to look pretty hopeless. It began to look insoluble. That wouldn't be unheard of, of course. Not by a long shot. A good many epidemiological problems are never fully solved. The Riverside outbreak I mentioned is one of them. They never found the ultimate source of the trouble. They never determined how S. typhimurium got into the water. Hospital outbreaks are particularly tricky. A bug can get into a hospital and practically defy detection. In a big hospital — in a hospital like the M. G. H., where you have over six thousand people employed — the pathways can be extremely complex. Everybody

I talked to was very consoling. They said I had an impossible problem. They said that I'd never run down the source, that nobody could run it down. I'd done everything that could be done, they said. That was true enough. At least, what I'd done was epidemiologically sound. The outbreak had been reported early on to the Massachusetts Department of Public Health, and Dr. Rubenstein — Daniel Rubenstein, the director of their Bureau of Hospital Facilities — had come over and reviewed our procedure and given it his approval. Another thing that my friends all said was that the outbreak seemed to be cooling off. It's probably burned itself out, they said. It's over. So relax. Forget it. They had a point about its cooling off. There hadn't been a new case since February 6. The old man in the Bulfinch Building was the last one. I tried to take their advice. I had plenty of other work to do at the hospital and in my laboratory and at Harvard. When the time came for me to make my report to the Infection Control Committee on February 23, I was almost convinced they were right.

"But they weren't. They could hardly have been more mistaken. On March 1, just six days after the meeting, Dr. Kunz's laboratory turned up another case. And that was merely No. 1 for the month. It was the first of a total of five. The first patient was in the White Building — on White Seven. He was a man of seventy-nine, and he had entered the hospital back in January with no presenting symptoms that in any way resembled those of salmonellosis. So his was clearly another hospital-acquired infection. So were those of No. 2 and No. 3 and No. 5. Case No. 4 was an infant on Burnham Five who had been cultured on arrival — in the emergency room. Case No. 2 was reported on March 16. He was a teen-age boy on White Five. The third came along on the following day — a nurse on Burnham Four. Then, on March 18, came No. 4. No. 5 was a teen-age girl on White Eleven. She turned up on March 19. Four cases in four days! I felt like throwing up my hands."

Dr. Kunz says: "And all in different places. It was like having a sniper up in a tower taking pot shots in every direction."

Dr. Lang says: "But then it really did cool off. March went out like a lamb. There were no more cases that month, and there were none in April and none in May. And there were none in the first half of June. I really thought it was over. A good thing, too. My wife was bloody sick of hearing about *S. cubana*, and for three months she got a relief. I didn't talk about it, but I didn't forget it. I put it out of the forefront of my mind and concentrated on my virus lab and on making rounds and on teaching, but I was too involved to give it up. It was my investigation, it was my responsibility — it was even more than that. It was my fascination. I never really gave up. I certainly never stopped running down possible leads. I think I must have known in my heart that this was just another hiatus.

"One idea I had was that the spread of the infection within the hospital might be attributable to sporadic carriers. It was obvious that the nurse on Burnham Four had been infected by one of her patients, and she could easily have carried the infection on to somebody else if our routine culturing hadn't picked her up. What I had in mind was hospital personnel that once in a while moved out of their regular bailiwick. Every now and then a nurse will special on another floor. Or a surgeon will answer a consultation in another building. And the X-ray people are always going somewhere. I checked up on everybody who had had any contact with any of the cases. That turned out to be a lot of people, and it took a lot of time, but it was no good. I drew a blank again. Another lead had to do with powdered milk. The National Communicable Disease Center of the U. S. Public Health Service puts out a monthly bulletin called *Salmonella Surveillance*, and the June issue had a report from the Oregon State Department of Health about two cases of *S. cubana* infection in infants that had been traced to contaminated instant nonfat dry milk. It was *S. cubana* that caught my eye, of course. But the vehicle was provocative, too. I began to think that I was finally on to something. Powdered milk or nutritives containing powdered milk are used extensively in hospitals. I went down and got out the charts and orders on our cases — and there it was. Powdered milk or some nutritive additive had been prescribed for practically all of them. I rounded up some samples of the various products and sent them down to Dr. Kunz. Then I got on the telephone to the manufacturer. And that was the end of that. I knew that the manufacturer had a reputation for maintaining a high standard of quality control, but I hadn't known just how careful they were until I talked to the plant. They told me that they cultured all their products before they shipped them out. And Dr. Kunz confirmed what they said. All of my samples were negative."

Dr. Kunz says: "We confirmed it, all right. But this thing was beginning to get on my nerves. We kept testing all this garbage that Dr. Lang kept sending down to the lab. We cultured every child that was discharged from Burnham. We cultured around three hundred hospital employees. We cultured God knows how much food and drugs. And the results were always the same. It didn't seem reasonable. *Cubana* ought to be showing up somewhere. I began to wonder if maybe we were doing something wrong."

Dr. Lang says: "It *was* a hiatus. The outbreak opened up again on June 15. That was a Wednesday. On Wednesday morning, Dr. Kunz called up to report another case, and that afternoon, he called me again and reported still another. They brought the grand total up to twenty. One of the new cases was a baby girl on Burnham Six, and the other was a man of thirty-nine on White Seven, and the records showed that both of them could have become infected only in the hospital. I ran around and gathered the same old information once again. I talked to the interns and the nurses and the residents. There was nothing else I could think to do, and, as always, it came to nothing. There was no link, no connection, no rational explanation. I met with Dr. Rubenstein. He and his department were giving us every kind of cooperation, but they were as stumped as we were. Dr. Kunz and I were beginning to think that what we needed was some help from the National Communicable Disease Center down in Atlanta. Their people have the training and the facilities to really dig into problems like this. But it wasn't up to us to ask them. The invitation would have to come from the State Health Department. And then we had another lull — another hiatus. It lasted exactly six weeks. It ended on July 26, a Wednesday, at about one-thirty in the afternoon.

"I had just got back from lunch and I was working in my office. The telephone rang and it was Dr. Kunz. We now had a total of twenty-one cases. His people had grown another culture of Group-G salmonella. The patient was another infant — a four-month-old boy. He had been a patient on Burnham Four since June 26, and the information was that his infection was hospital-acquired. I hung up and sat back and looked at my notes. Then I went and had a talk with Dr. Mort Swartz. He's our chief of clinical infectious disease. And I don't know, but we got to thinking that here was an opportunity for a really special study. This little boy was an isolated case — the first new case in weeks. He was a crib child and therefore not very mobile — no wandering around or playing with other kids. And, if only because of his age, his diet would be relatively simple. So I went up on the floor. I started with his chart. It didn't tell me much. He had been admitted to the hospital with a general diagnosis of failure to thrive. Since then he had lost weight, and on July 24 he had developed diarrhea. His condition now was fair. I went over to the floor nurse's desk and got out the order book. An order book is a record of the physician's specific instructions for the care of the patient. It covers medication, diet, tests — everything. I found the boy's page, and read through the entries. There was a request to check on vital signs every four hours, and a diet warning about a possible milk allergy. Diet was limited to strained foods and meats, and to two supplements — d-xylose, a nonfermenting sugar used in a test procedure, and a milk substitute called Nutramigen. Two drugs were prescribed — a multiple-vitamin preparation and an oral iron preparation. There was an order for a urinalysis, and for four stool tests. The stool tests were a test for fat and fibers, a test for trypsin-enzyme activity, a routine culture for pathogens, and a carmine-dye transit time test. All the tests had been done — the stool-culture request was obviously the source of Dr. Kunz's salmonella report. But what interested me was the use of carmine dye. That lit me up like a light bulb. I don't know why exactly. It made me think of the Santa Claus specimen, but we had ruled that out of the picture. I think it was just the coincidence. I had hardly even heard of carmine dye until the Santa Claus case, and here it was again. That was enough to arouse my curiosity.

"I got a nurse to open the medication closet, and I took samples of everything the boy had been given — d-xylose, Nutramigen, vitamins, oral iron, carmine dye. The first information I wanted was what these drugs contained and how they were made. I carried my samples down to the pharmacy in the Burnham basement and showed them to the chief of pharmacy and his assistant. When they came to the carmine dye, they looked at the capsules and said it came from a manufacturer of synthetic dyes. My heart sank down to my heels. Synthetic products don't usually harbor Salmonellae. They inhibit the growth of bacteria. I asked if carmine was an aniline dye. The chief wasn't sure, but his assistant had been around a long time, and he said he didn't think so. Carmine was made from something called cochineal. The chief got out a copy of the 'Merck Index' and looked up carmine dye. The other pharmacist was right. It defined carmine as a pigment made from dried cochineal. But what was cochineal? The chief went back and got a copy of 'The Dispensatory of the United States of America,' and we looked it up in that."

The entry reads: "Cochineal consists of dried female insects, *Coccus cacti* Linné (Fam. *Coccidae*), enclosing the young larvae. U. S. P. The B. P. definition differs in giving the name of this insect as *Dactylopius coccus* Costa and specifying that it contain eggs as well as larvae. The cochineal insect is indigenous to Mexico, Peru, and Central America, and in general appearance resembles a wood louse. The red dye found in the remains of the female insect has long been esteemed by the old races in these subtropical countries. Indeed, not only did they appreciate its value, but in order to increase the supplies, the cacti with the insects were successfully cultivated many years before even Cortez landed in Mexico in the early part of the sixteenth century. . . . The insect feeds upon various species of the *Cactaceae*. It has spread into other parts of South and Central America and has been introduced into the West Indies, East Indies, Canary Islands, Southern Spain, and Algeria. The cultivation of cochineal is rather simple in a tropical climate; all that is necessary is to have the cochineal insects and the proper cacti. . . . The insects are 'sown' on the cacti in the open fields, where fecundation takes place. After this, the females attach themselves to the plant, and when their bodies have become swollen from the development of the enormous number of eggs, they are scraped off and killed either by boiling water or by the fumes of burning sulfur. . . . Powdered cochineal is very dusky to very dark red. It contains fragments of muscle fibers; portions of the chitinous epidermis with wax glands; fragments of larvae with coiled proboscides; occasional claws and segments of the legs; and fragments of antennae. . . . During 1952, a total of 83,713 pounds of cochineal was imported into this country from the Canary Islands, Peru, and Chile. . . . Cochineal was at one time supposed by some to possess anodyne properties, and used in whooping cough and neuralgia. At present, it is employed only as a coloring agent."

Dr. Lang says: "That really lit me up. I knew I had found the explanation. I was sure of it. There were two particular points. One was that carmine dye is ground-up insects. What could be a better vehicle than that? The other was that the insect is indigenous to Central America. I know it's ridiculous but I saw an association. Central America. Cuba. *Cubana*. I thanked the pharmacists and gathered up my samples and carried them over to Dr. Kunz's office."

Dr. Kunz says: "Ground-up insects — it seemed possible. I wasn't really excited. We had been through so many dry runs. I just for the first time wasn't bored to tears. But I turned everything except the carmine over to the girls. I planted the carmine myself. And it was the only sample that grew anything. I planted it on August 1, and on August 3 it grew a culture that tested out as Group-G salmonella."

Dr. Lang says: "That was good enough for me. I didn't wait for the New York Salmonella Center to identify the serotype as *S. cubana*. Which it did, of course, toward the end of the following week. We knew that the carmine dye was contaminated. But that didn't solve the problem unless the *cubana* patients and carmine could be linked. There were fifteen hospital-acquired cases in addition to the little boy on Burnham Four. I found that carmine-dye tests had been prescribed for eleven of them. The four other hospital cases were no embarrassment. One of the four was the Burnham nurse, and her infection had almost certainly come from one of her patients. As for the others, the fact that carmine wasn't noted in the orders didn't really mean a thing. I was willing to assume that they had been given carmine. Or they could be secondary cases. I assumed it from their histories. They all appeared to be suffering from some sort of gastrointestinal dysfunction, and carmine isn't always entered in the orders. It isn't required to be, because it isn't a medicine or what we call a charge drug — a drug for which the patient is charged.

"It took a little longer to explain the five infections that must have been acquired outside the hospital. One thing that had to be clarified first was the nature of the carmine contamination. Carmine dye is dispensed at the M. G. H. in capsules that are filled here at the hospital. Could the carmine have been contaminated in the course of that operation? Dr. Kunz got the answer to that by culturing carmine from the sealed jars in which it reached the hospital. To be absolutely sure of his results, he made his tests in the sterile room in my virus laboratory, where I do tissue cultures. There was no possibility there of any outside contamination. Well, the carmine from the sealed jars grew *S. cubana.* That naturally raised the question of the other local hospitals. They used carmine, too. Why hadn't they been getting any *cubana* infections? Dr. Rubenstein and his associates at the Massachusetts Department of Public Health were able to suggest an answer to that. They turned the answer up in the course of an intensive investigation they mounted as soon as they got our carmine-dye report. They found the explanation in the hospitals' laboratory procedures. The usual approach to salmonella detection in those laboratories was serologic, but their diagnostic antisera embraced only Groups A through E. A Group-G salmonella could escape detection. It wouldn't even be recognized as a salmonella. So it was entirely possible that our twenty-one cases of *S. cubana* were not the only cases in town. They were merely the only cases diagnosed as such. But how did our outside cases get their infections? My answer is only a guess — it couldn't be anything else — but I'm inclined to think it's the truth. Our experience set in motion a series of investigations by various state and federal agencies. The Communicable Disease Center and the Food and Drug Administration were particularly active. They found carmine dye contaminated with *S. cubana* throughout the country, and several outbreaks identical with ours. There was only one manufacturer of carmine dye in the United States, and all of his stock was contaminated. At that point, of course, the sale of carmine was halted, and all hospitals and other users warned about its dangers. They also found that the use of carmine dye was not limited to hospitals — or even to medicine. It was also used as a coloring agent in numerous foods and drugs. The investigation showed that the American manufacturer sold carmine — directly or through distributors — to twenty-eight food companies, ten spice companies, thirty-three pharmaceutical companies, seven cosmetic companies, and fifty-six less specialized companies, and the contaminated products they found included candy, chewing gum, preservatives, seasonings, meat, ice cream, and tomato extracts. Incidentally, the presence of carmine dye in these products was not noted on the label. The labeling law applies only to *artificial* coloring agents. Well, I think that answers the question. Not every person exposed to salmonella gets sick, but those cases of ours were highly susceptible people. I mean, they were already sick."

Dr. Kunz says: "We had an explanation for everything except my Santa Claus specimen. I think I can explain how the original specimen was contaminated. Carmine dye was not one of its ingredients, but it was the main ingredient of the blood sample that the jokers also made. I talked to them again, and it seems probable that a swab that was used to stir the blood specimen was later used to stir the other specimen. So there *was* a certain amount of carmine in the original Santa Claus specimen. But there was much more carmine in my reconstructed specimen, and yet that culture was negative. I don't know why. Maybe the carmine I used was the last of an earlier, uncontaminated supply. I don't know. I can't explain it. It's inexplicable."

The case was closed at the September meeting of the Committee on Infection Control. The secretary's account of that portion of the meeting read: "A follow-up report on Salmonella was presented by Dr. Lang, who reviewed the investigation within the hospital and in conjunction with the F.D.A. and the C.D.C. The source of hospital-acquired *Salmonella cubana* was traced to carmine red, which has been discontinued for clinical use. Mr. Webb is to circulate a statement to the staff regarding the discontinuance of carmine red, and he awaits direction from the F.D.A. on how to process the stock on hand. The Committee feels that to sterilize the present stock is perhaps hazardous, and that it should be discarded. At the moment, carbon is being used as a substitute for carmine red."

The conclusion of the investigation at the Massachusetts General Hospital was not quite the end of the matter. There remained the question of how the carmine dye had become contaminated. The natural assumption was that the contamination occurred in the course of processing at the plant of the American manufacturer. An early finding by the government investigators seemed to confirm that supposition. They found that although the manufacture of carmine dye included three processes employing heat (leaching, precipitation, and drying), the heat employed was seldom enough to destroy a salmonella. Another finding, however, suggested another explanation. A bacteriological examination revealed that recently imported stocks of dried cochineal at the plant were crawling with *S. cubana*. It thus seemed possible that the insect *Dactylopius coccus* was itself the source of the contamination, and this baleful possibility was presently supported by word of similar findings at the plants of the leading manufacturers in Britain and in West Germany. It was also determined that all of these manufacturers — American, British, and German — were supplied by dealers in both Peru and the Canary Islands.

The entomological implications of these revelations changed the course of the investigation. They moved it from the national to the international scene. In June 1967, two CDC investigators — Steven A. Schroeder and Ariel Thomson — were dispatched to Peru to make a thorough study of the cochineal industry there. Dr. Lang and Dr. Kunz were invited to make a similar study in the Canary Islands. They accepted the assignment, and carried it out in August. The results of the two field studies were summarized by Dr. Schroeder in a subsequent report.

His conclusion read: "In Peru and in some areas of the Canary Islands, the cochineal insect grows wild on cactuses . . . while in parts of the Canary Islands, there are actual plantations where the insects are cultivated. The insects mature during the dry season, and in Peru are harvested by Indians, who then sell the insects to local merchants. The merchants spread the insects on canvas cloths and allow them to sun dry on the streets or in yards, often adjacent to animal feces and flies. After a week or so of drying, the insects are put into sacks or tin cans and are sold at irregular intervals to brokers for the three or four large Peruvian cochineal exporting firms. . . . Dr. Thomson and I collected numerous samples of insects on cactuses, insects prior to being dried, while drying, and after drying. Of the more than fifty samples analyzed, only two, both of dried insects, were positive for salmonellae. The serotypes identified were *S. newport* and *S. enteritidis*, both of which are quite common throughout the world. Similarly, Drs. Kunz and Lang examined twelve samples from the Canary

93

Islands, all of which were negative for salmonellae. It would appear therefore that salmonellae are not intrinsic to the cochineal insect, but are introduced, possibly through fecal exposure during the drying process. It seems reasonable to speculate that a batch of insects containing *S. cubana* contaminated machinery used in carmine-dye production, resulting in continuing contamination of the dye product with this same serotype. . . . Terminal heat sterilization [in processing] seems to have eliminated the salmonella hazard of carmine dye."

# In the Bughouse

One of the continuing perplexities of medicine is the nature of epidemics. The epidemic diseases themselves are no longer much of a mystery. Their causes (microbial, fungal, metazoal), their modes of transmission (by respiration, by ingestion, by insect or animal bite), and the means of controlling their spread (immunization, sanitation, isolation) have all been pretty well established. What still remains to be fathomed is the dynamics of the interplay of pathogenic virulence and human susceptibility that determines their comings and goings. It is not yet known just why certain diseases will suddenly appear, rapidly proliferate, and gradually peter out, and then — two years or three years or five years later — as suddenly reappear. It is also unclear just why, as sometimes happens, a disease will simply vanish.

There are several such disappearances reliably on record. Those of leprosy (which ravaged Europe as a plague of pandemic proportions in the thirteenth and fourteenth centuries, and then, in the early sixteenth century, spontaneously withdrew to its native Asia and Africa) and a frequently fatal complex of high fever, prostration, and ubiquitous aches and pains called the sweating sickness (which made five epidemic appearances in England between 1485 and 1551, and has never been heard of there, or anywhere, again) are among the most notorious. Others include scarlet fever (which, after several centuries of epidemic vigor and violence, transformed itself in the nineteen-forties into a generally innocuous disease of almost total immobility), von Economo's encephalitis (which was first described in Rumania in 1915, blazed its way around the world for a decade, and vanished in 1926), and the incomparably savage species of influenza whose only documented visitation was the worldwide epidemic of 1918-19. A more recent member of this fugitive company is a cosmopolitan curiosity variously known as Akureyri disease, benign myalgic encephalomyelitis, epidemic vegetative neuritis, Iceland disease, acute infective encephalomyelitis, atypical poliomyelitis, and epidemic neuromyasthenia. The last of these is the name most epidemiologists prefer.

Epidemic neuromyasthenia, as its name proclaims, is an epidemic disease whose more conspicuous clinical manifestations include a derangement of the nervous system (neuro) and muscular (my) weakness (asthenia). It was first recognized as an entity in Iceland in 1948. In the fall of that year, an epidemic of what appeared to be poliomyelitis broke out in Akureyri, Iceland's second-largest city, and when it finally ended, some four months later, a total of four hundred and sixty-five cases had been reported. An inquiry undertaken early in the outbreak by a team of public-health investigators under Björn Sigurdsson, director of the Institute for Experimental Pathology at the University of Iceland, at once eliminated poliomyelitis as the probable cause of the trouble. In fact, Sigurdsson and his associates noted in a report published in the *American Journal of Hygiene* in 1950, "The clinical and epidemiological characteristics of the Akureyri disease . . . do not fit in well with any of the epidemic diseases with which we are familiar." They then described its several peculiarities: "This disease was characterized by pains in the nape and back, accompanied by fever that was usually low. Paresthesias and hyperesthesias [extremes of skin sensitivity] were common, and approximately 28 percent of the patients showed muscular paresis [an incomplete paralysis] that usually was light, but in a few cases very severe, and could hardly be distinguished from regular poliomyelitis. The disease, in some cases, ran a rather chronic course in that the fever sometimes lasted for several weeks, and relapses of fever, paresis, and sensibility disturbances were noticed in several instances some weeks after the initial attack. Even the slightest physical exertion or exposure to cold during the earlier stages of illness tended to aggravate the symptoms and bring on new manifestations of the disease. . . . Disturbances such as nervousness, sleeplessness, and loss of memory were rather common complaints after this disease in otherwise normal persons many months after the acute attack." In addition, the investigators pointed out, the Akureyri disease, unlike poliomyelitis, which has a predilection for the very young (most adolescents and adults having acquired a certain immunity), took the great majority of its victims from the teens and twenties, and — as a further distinction from poliomyelitis — none of the cases was fatal. A final reason for supposing the existence of a new disease was provided by the laboratory. Blood and other material taken from patients at various stages of illness were tested for evidence of poliomyelitis and a number of other possibilities — Coxsackie-virus infection, influenza (three strains), equine encephalomyelitis (two strains), St. Louis encephalitis, Japanese B. encephalitis, rabies, choriomeningitis, and Q fever. All the tests were negative.

Sigurdsson's supposition that the disease he and his associates encountered in Akureyri was a new one has been amply confirmed by time. In the fifteen years since their ambiguous find was introduced to medicine in the pages of the *American Journal of Hygiene*, some twenty outbreaks of a disease closely answering its description have been reported in seven widely scattered countries — Australia, Denmark, England, Germany, Greece, the Union of South Africa, and the United States. Time has also shown, however, that the appearance of epidemic neuromyasthenia in Akureyri in 1948 was probably not its first appearance. It was merely the first appearance at which it was confidently recognized as something new and different. Most investigators are now persuaded that its distinctive features can be plainly discerned in at least three earlier epidemic episodes.

The first of these occurred in 1934 in Los Angeles, and affected one hundred ninety-eight people. All the victims were employees of the Los Angeles County General Hospital, most of them were nurses, and all of them recovered. An investigation of the outbreak was conducted by an assistant surgeon of the United States Public Health Service named A. G. Gilliam, and he recorded his findings in a report somewhat equivocally

98

entitled "Epidemiological Study of an Epidemic, Diagnosed as Poliomyelitis, Occurring Among the Personnel of the Los Angeles County General Hospital During the Summer of 1934." The tone of Gilliam's title reflected that of his report. "Coincidentally with an epidemic of poliomyelitis in the City and County of Los Angeles, Calif. in the summer of 1934, there occurred among the employees of the Los Angeles County General Hospital an epidemic of illness diagnosed at the time as poliomyelitis," he observed in an introductory note. "If this diagnosis may be accepted in any large proportion of the cases, the epidemic is unique in the history of poliomyelitis because of the altogether unusual symptomatology and the extraordinarily high attack rate in an adult population. If the disease was not poliomyelitis, the epidemic is equally extraordinary in presenting a clinical and epidemiological picture which, so far as is known, is without parallel." Gilliam's report included thirty-two detailed clinical portraits, and the reasons for his uncertainty are apparent in any and all of them. Case No. 131 ("W. F., 27, attendant") reads:

On June 18 [the patient] developed a peculiar, diffuse headache which was not particularly severe, was nauseated and felt generally "rotten" and extremely restless. There was also moderately severe pain along the ulnar distribution of both arms and in both thumbs. The following day her neck and back were definitely stiff. While working, she found that her arms were generally weak and she could hardly lift a baby or carry a tray, so she was admitted to the hospital. Physical examination confirmed the stiff neck and back and also discovered tenderness in the right deltoid, biceps, and right thigh. The temperature was 99.4° (the highest during this hospitalization). . . . The patient vomited after admission. On June 20, orthopedic examination revealed "numerous muscle groups weak or tender"; she was placed on a Bradford frame with all extremities immobilized. . . . She stated she was

99

delirious during the day. . . . About June 24, severe muscle twitching, cramps, and pain developed, and lasted 10 days. She also had peculiar position sensations: "the feet felt like they were clear across the room" and she "couldn't wriggle the toes"; when "the eyes were closed, I felt like I was falling." Orthopedic note states on June 29, "muscles of the left arm normal; lower extremities tender; muscles right arm still tender." . . . Routine physiotherapy muscle tests being completely normal on July 12 and July 19, the patient was discharged on the latter date. Following her discharge, she had repeated episodes of terrific headache, fever, chills, vomiting, general aches and pains, and stiff neck, and she spent most of the time in bed at home. On September 18 she was readmitted, because, in addition to the general symptoms, she developed painful, burning urination. Her temperature had been recorded on the outside as 101° but the highest while hospitalized was 100°. No muscle weakness was detected on careful muscle check, but hospitalization was continued until October 30 because of intermittent headache, pain, general malaise, and nervousness. Following discharge, she had frequent insomnia, headache, and nervousness, and easy fatigue and calf pain after exertion. These symptoms gradually disappeared and she was considered able to return to duty on December 30.

Gilliam was nevertheless inspired to end his report on a somewhat more positive note. "Despite the peculiar clinical character of many of these cases," he wrote, "there appear to be good grounds for assuming that the majority of them resulted from infection with the virus of poliomyelitis."

The other earlier outbreaks that hindsight has identified as epidemic neuromyasthenia occurred near Fond du Lac, Wisconsin, in 1936, and in Harefield, England, in 1939. The scene of the Fond du Lac outbreak was a Roman Catholic convent, and thirty-five girls between the ages of fourteen and twenty-one were involved, all of them novices or postulants. The cause of the trouble was thought at first to be some form of encephalitis, and the United States Public Health Service was so informed. The symptoms, as reported to the Surgeon General by a Public Health Service investigator named Charles A. Armstrong, were rich and varied — chills and fever, headache, sore throat, pain in the back and chest, sweating of the hands and feet, tingling in the hands and feet, leg pain, difficulty in moving the legs, ringing in the ears, dizziness, confusion, apathy — but the picture they presented was diagnostically opaque. Armstrong could find no convincing evidence of encephalitis or of any other disease he knew, and he frankly acknowledged defeat: "The condition . . . is not explainable on the basis of any infection or intoxication with which I am familiar." The Harefield outbreak occurred in a hospital — the Harefield Sanatorium — and it felled a total of seven. All were women, all were young, all were nurses. Their complaints included fatigue, sore throat, muscular aches and pains, paresis, muscle cramps, nausea, urinary retention, depression, and nervous tension. As usual, they all recovered. In a report to the *Lancet*, entitled "Persistent Myalgia Following Sore Throat," two members of the sanatorium staff attributed the outbreak to "an unidentified virus."

The exhumation of these early outbreaks does more than simply swell the list of the probable appearances of epidemic neuromyasthenia. It serves to further document two singular aspects of the disease. One, of course, is its striking predilection for young women. The other is its almost equally striking predilection for closed, or cloistered, communities. Of twenty-four accepted outbreaks of epidemic neuromyasthenia, ten have occurred in hospitals and among hospital personnel, one (at Fond du Lac) in a convent, and one (in Germany) in an army barracks, and in many of the others there were doctors and nurses among the victims. Thirty-four of the four hundred sixty-five victims in Akureyri were students at a boarding school.

Ten epidemics of epidemic neuromyasthenia have been reliably recorded in the United States since its discovery at Akureyri. They have ranged in size from an outbreak of seven cases (in Pittsfield and Williamstown, Massachusetts, in 1956) to an explosion (in Tallahassee, Florida, in 1954) that totaled four hundred fifty. The first of the ten (nineteen cases, fifteen of them young women) occurred in Alexandria Bay, in northern New York, in the late summer of 1950, or only a few weeks after the publication of the Akureyri study. Its resemblance to the disease described by Sigurdsson and his associates was almost immediately apparent, and this prompted two physicians of the area — D. Naldrett White and Robert B. Burtch — to write an account of the visitation. Their paper, entitled "Iceland Disease: A New Infection Simulating Acute Anterior Poliomyelitis," appeared in *Neurology* in 1954, and was the first corroborative celebration of Sigurdsson's discovery. The most recent American outbreak of any considerable size occurred at Punta Gorda, Florida, in 1956. It is also the only one of any considerable size that the United States Public Health Service has had an opportunity to investigate thoroughly.

The Punta Gorda epidemic came to the attention of the United States Public Health Service by way of a request for help from an epidemiologist on the staff of the Florida State Board of Health named James Bond. His request, as is customary in such cases, was addressed to the chief of the Epidemic Intelligence Service at the Communicable Disease Center of the USPHS, in Atlanta. In 1956, that was Donald A.

Henderson. Dr. Henderson (now an executive of the Epidemiology Program at the CDC) found it on his desk on the morning of Wednesday, May 9.

"Dr. Bond's letter didn't tell us very much," Dr. Henderson says. "It was just a note. He was reporting sixty-four cases of what he called Iceland disease. The term 'epidemic neuromyasthenia' hadn't yet come into general use. The outbreak had begun in the early part of March, and he had been on the scene for about a week. He would be grateful for any advice or assistance we might be able to give him. That was about the gist of it. But it was quite enough to arouse my interest. I'd never seen a case of epidemic neuromyasthenia, but I knew about it. I'd read the literature. And I knew that Bond knew what he was talking about. He'd been in on the big outbreak of epidemic neuromyasthenia down in Tallahassee a couple of years before. So I put in a call to Bond at his office in Jacksonville. We had a little talk, and he told me what he could. All but one of the cases were women — white women — and their ages ranged from thirty to sixty. The other case was a seventy-year-old man — also white. Punta Gorda was a predominantly white community. It had a population of around three thousand, only about five hundred of them Negroes. The town was situated on the southwest coast, on Charlotte Harbor, and was the seat of Charlotte County. It was a shrimp-fishing port, with some farms and cattle ranches inland, and it drew a few vacationers in the winter. It had a twenty-three-bed hospital and three practicing physicians, and it was on their appeal that Bond had come into the case. The clinical picture was almost exactly what he had seen in the Tallahassee outbreak. The principal presenting symptoms were recurrent sharp pains in the muscles of the back and neck, severe headache, disturbances of coordination, and some transient motor and sensory dysfunctions. Plus a strong emotional overlay — tension, anxiety, depression. The physical findings were essentially unimportant, and the results of certain routine laboratory tests had all been within the normal range. At the moment, the situation was stable — no new cases in almost a week. Well, that suggested that maybe the outbreak was waning. If so, there was no particular hurry about our getting down there, since the best time to carry out an investigation is during the acute epidemic phase. When that phase has passed, time is not of critical importance. I was disappointed, of course, but I was also rather relieved. An immediate investigation would have imposed a bit of a strain. We were very shorthanded right then, and our annual Epidemic Intelligence Service conference was coming up in a couple of weeks. So I proposed a visit in June. Bond thought that would do very well. Meanwhile, he said, he would keep me in touch with developments.

"Which he did. And very promptly. I got a call from Bond the following week — the following Wednesday, in fact. The wane had turned out to be only a lull. Five new cases had just been reported. He thought we might want to make a change in our plans. The best I could manage was a compromise. We were still shorthanded, but no longer desperately so. I had an investigator more or less available — a young EIS physician named David C. Poskanzer. I said I would get him off as quickly as possible. I got him off on Sunday, and he was down in Punta Gorda most of the week. That was the week before the EIS conference. Poskanzer returned to Atlanta on Friday, and his report was a feature of the meeting. One thing that particularly struck him about the disease was its enormous and confusing array of symptoms. They were protean — absolutely protean. He stressed that over and over again. I thought I knew what he meant. That is, the point had been emphasized in all the literature I'd read. But I was mistaken. The symptomatology of epidemic neuromyasthenia is extremely hard to picture. You really have to see it for yourself.

"Well, I got to see it a few days later. Once the conference was out of the way, I was free to recruit a team for a real investigation — a comprehensive clinical and epidemiological study. I didn't need an army. I knew from Bond and Poskanzer that we could count on a lot of local help. The team I picked consisted of Poskanzer and me and two others. They were E. Charles Kunkle, a professor of neurology at Duke University School of Medicine who also serves as a Public Health Service consultant, and Seymour S. Kalter, the chief of the diagnostic-methodology unit of the virus-and-rickettsia section of our Laboratory Branch. Kalter, Poskanzer, Kunkle, and I got to Punta Gorda on Sunday, May 27, and checked into a motel that Poskanzer knew about. Then we had a meeting with Bond and the local physicians, and on Monday morning we got to work. We stayed at Punta Gorda four days — through Thursday. That was our first visit. One of the characteristics of epidemic neuromyasthenia is a prolonged and relapsing course. We learned that early on. A patient seems to shake it off, and then it comes back again. So we made two followup visits to see it through to the end. We returned for two days in October, and again, for another two days, in November of the following year.

"I think, on the whole, the study was worth the time and effort. It was well worth it. All the same, it was a bit maddening. We learned everything, and nothing. The point is, though, we had everything *to* learn. We were up against a new disease, and essentially still a completely mysterious one. The literature — the earlier studies — hadn't done much more than establish it as an entity. That gave our investigation a very special character. Diagnosis is the key in most investigations. Once that is accomplished, the rest is usually only a matter of time. The cause is implicit in the nature of the disease, and the cause suggests the source of the trouble. It tells us what to look for and where. In this case, we had a diagnosis — a kind of diagnosis — but it told us hardly anything. It was only a name — a label. We had to begin at the absolute bottom. First of all, we had to examine the diagnosis. We had to determine whether a specific disease entity was actually present in epidemic form. That involved the phenomenon that Poskanzer had stressed at the conference — the enormous and confusing array of symptoms. The significant symptoms had to be determined and the clinical picture clearly defined. Then we had to determine the scope of the outbreak. The next step was to determine the cause and the source of the trouble.

"Nobody seriously questioned the presence of an epidemic in Punta Gorda. The local medical records showed that, beginning around the end of February, a gradually increasing number of mostly women patients had been observed and hospitalized with a complex of more or less prostrating symptoms that seemed to fit the entity we now call epidemic neuromyasthenia. There was a total of sixty-nine such patients on record at the time of our arrival. About thirty of them were still sick, and from that group we selected twenty-one cases — seventeen women and four men — for definitive clinical analysis. At the same time, with the help of neighborhood volunteers, we organized a house-to-house survey in order to get a clearer notion of the actual incidence and distribution of the illness.

Medical records are only an indication of the scope of an epidemic. There are always a number of victims who can't or won't see a doctor. This was particularly true in Punta Gorda. Our interviewers visited nearly four hundred homes and talked to more than a thousand people, and they turned up sixty-two additional cases. They were very definitely cases, too. The interviewers accepted as cases only those that met a fairly rigid set of criteria. These criteria were our own, developed from our preliminary clinical findings, and they established three diagnostic points. A definite change in physical or emotional status, or both, indicating an onset of illness — that was the first criterion. The second was an illness of at least seven days. The third was the presence of at least six out of nine relevant symptoms of recent occurrence or exacerbation. They were fatigue, neck pain, headache, aching-limb pain, loss of appetite, nausea, impairment of memory, depression, and paresthesia. I was in on several of the interviews, and I can testify that we managed to get the facts — one way or another. I remember one case in point. It was a preacher — white, middle-aged, and married. His wife had been eliminated — no significant symptoms — but we weren't quite sure about him. He had been sick, and his symptoms were generally provocative. Except on the emotional side. He insisted that there was nothing wrong with his mind or his memory. As we rose to go, the interviewer asked him if she could have a glass of water. Of course, he said, and left the room. But almost at once he was back. The interviewer had asked him for something — what was it? She told him. Oh, yes. He started out of the room again, and then stopped and called upstairs to his wife. Where did they keep the ice cubes? She told him, and he went on out to the kitchen. But a moment later he called her again. This time he wanted to know just how many cubes should go in the glass. We added him to the case list.

"I called our criteria fairly rigid. That's all they were, I'm afraid. They were as rigid as we could possibly make them, and I think they were reasonably effective, but they fell a bit short of scientific excellence. Epidemic neuromyasthenia is a most ungrateful disease in that respect. Its manifestations are subjective rather than objective. It produces all kinds of symptoms but — to the best of our present knowledge — very few signs. That was the first and possibly the most important thing we learned from our twenty-one detailed clinical studies. There was practically nothing that we could see or touch or measure. I mean, there were no lesions to examine, no big livers or tender spleens to feel, no jaundice, no classically paralyzed limbs, no cloudy chest X-rays, no laboratory data to analyze. We used to sit in my room at the motel after dinner and puzzle it over and over. None of us had ever seen anything like it. We just couldn't put it together. It was bizarre. Even the signs that did turn up were fantastic. Most of the patients complained of paresthesia — areas of decreased or increased skin sensitivity. They could generally guide us to the specific patch, and when the patch was on the back — out of the patient's sight — we always marked it in color. The next day, we would question the patient again, and invariably he guided us to a different — an unmarked — area. But the curious thing was that none of the areas encompassed by these paresthesias correspond to any recognized area innervated by a nerve or nerves. One woman patient complained of nodules on her arms. We looked where she told us to look, but there was nothing there that we could see or feel — no sign of any kind of lump. That's funny, she said, they *were* there. She said she knew because the site was still tender. We humored her. We asked her to let us know if and when another nodule appeared, and we went on to the next examination. She called us the very next day. She had another nodule. We trotted around to her room, and — holy Christmas! She was right. She did have a nodule. In fact, there were two of them — little pea-sized swellings on the underside of her left wrist. There was no discoloration, but they were sensitive to the touch. Or so she said. Well, this was getting interesting. It seemed possible that we were on to something that the laboratory could test and maybe identify. We persuaded her to let us take a sliver of one of the nodules for a biopsy examination, and one of the hospital staff came in and did the job. But, oh dear! — he didn't go deep enough, and nothing showed up. That was a crushing defeat. It was maddening. Bescause that was the end of her nodules. They never came back. I tell you, we began to feel that we were living in the bughouse.

"The bughouse possibility actually occurred to us. We simply couldn't put together a pathophysiological explanation. We got no help from the laboratory, and the results of our physical examinations were just as useless. That left us with nothing to go on but the histories — what the patients themselves could tell us. And the more of their complaints we heard, the more we began to wonder about a functional explanation. So many of the symptoms were psychoneurotic symptoms. I'll give you an example — a more or less typical case. She was a young unmarried woman, a beautician by trade, and one of our twenty-one closely studied cases. The course of her illness was especially characteristic. It came on quite insidiously toward the end of April. There was a gradual onset of fatigue, accompanied by intermittent headache and neck pain.

At about the same time, she became aware of a peculiar sensation in her right leg. It felt numb and weak, and every now and then she seemed to stumble. She began to feel clumsy at her work, and her hands began to shake. It got harder and harder for her to write. Then her memory began to fail. She would forget the names of her regular customers, and she couldn't remember what to charge for the various regular services. That went on for about a month. Then, suddenly, her headache and neck pain increased in severity, and she developed a crippling backache. Her headache was practically prostrating. So she went to see a doctor. She described the symptoms I've mentioned, and added that she felt as if she were shaking all over inside. Four days later, she developed diarrhea, nausea and vomiting, and vertigo, and was hospitalized. She remained in the hospital a month. During that time, she complained of a feeling of choking, difficulty in swallowing, and hyperventilation — the feeling of being unable to take a deep breath. She complained of pain around her eyes and intermittent double vision. There were times when it seemed to her that her heart doubled or tripled its beat. She constantly complained of fatigue and depression, and she often cried without provocation. She also complained of swellings in her arms and legs, her abdomen, and her face, but there was no objective evidence of this. Nor was there any apparent explanation of her trouble in swallowing or in taking a deep breath, and there was no electrocardiographic confirmation of her accelerated heartbeat. The only positive physical finding was tenderness in two small areas in her back. She was given aspirin for her headache and other pains, but it didn't seem to do much good. Around the end of June, she began to improve, and she was discharged to convalesce at home. We got the next installment of the story when we saw her again in October. For about a week after her discharge, she seemed to be almost well. And then she had a relapse. All her symptoms recurred, and she was laid up in bed at home for three weeks. In August, she again felt better, and returned to work. Her headaches and neck pains continued intermittently, and the slightest exertion exhausted her. She needed at least ten hours of sleep every night, and she took a nap every afternoon. Her most disabling complaint, however, was depression. She was still depressed when we saw her that October, and her mind was conspicuously slowed. She was unable to perform various simple tests — repeating a set of five numbers in reverse, or subtracting serially from one hundred. There was also still some tenderness in her back, and we noted a slight insensitivity to pain in her lower right leg. Her difficulties in mentation were a bit equivocal. This was true, of course, in most of the other cases, too. We had no basis for comparison. It was quite possible that her memory was normally bad. And maybe she was just naturally a bit thick in the head. But the third visit cleared that up. When we saw her in November of the following year, she was fully herself again. And she was a conspicuously bright young woman.

"You can see why the possibility of a psychoneurotic explanation came so readily to mind. Every symptom that poor woman had was conceivably psychogenic, and the same was true of the symptoms of all the other cases. Depression. Terrifying dreams. Crying without provocation. Nausea and headache and diarrhea. Back and neck pains. Imaginary fever. Problems of memory and mentation. Vertigo. Hyperventilation. Menstrual irregularities. Difficulty in swallowing. Fatigue. Fast heart. Imaginary swellings. Paresthesia. And paresis. But paresis of a very curious sort — an unwillingness, rather than an inability, to move an arm or a leg. Almost a fear of movement. It was like a hysterical paralysis. But there are no waves or epidemics of hysterical paralysis. They simply don't happen. And that was the trouble with a psychoneurotic explanation of the epidemic. There were plenty of psychoneurotic symptoms, but they weren't enough in themselves to support a mass-reaction hypothesis. There was, in fact, every objection to such an explanation. For one thing, so far as we could discover, nothing had happened in Punta Gorda that could have excited a mass reaction. For another, the separate illnesses appeared at scattered intervals. That was clearly spelled out in the histories of both the reported cases and those we turned up in the house-to-house survey. The illnesses were scattered all the way from February to June. Moreover — and this is most significant — there was hardly a ripple of apprehension among the general population of the town. Nobody even suggested that the schools be closed. Or the movies or the beaches or anything. Nobody seemed in the least alarmed by what was going on. It was just the reverse of a panic situation.

"So we dropped the bughouse theory. But if it wasn't a question of mass-reaction hysteria, what *was* the anatomy of the epidemic? We went to work on the possible sources of trouble. Could it be something transmitted by insects? Most of the recorded outbreaks of epidemic neuromyasthenia had occurred in the insect season. But the answer here was no. There had been few mosquitoes or any other possible insect vectors in Punta Gorda until the second half of April, and the epidemic was well under way by then. We checked the usual urban sources of mass illness — the drinking water, the milk, the general food supply, the beaches. The answer again was negative. There wasn't a hint of contamination anywhere. We considered the possibility of a toxic product of some sort. We searched the case histories for some provocative coincidence — the common use of a certain cosmetic or household chemical. But nothing came of that, either. There weren't any likely links. There was no single factor of any kind uniquely common to the group affected. The only kind of coincidence we found was one for which the literature had rather explicitly prepared us. That was a disproportionately high rate of illness among hospital and medical personnel. The attack rate for the general adult population was around six percent — which, by the way, is quite high. But it was *forty-two* percent for the hospital and medical people. Sixteen of a total of thirty-eight doctors, nurses, technicians, and hospital receptionists, cooks, maids, and janitors were on our roll of cases.

"We left with one possibility. It was also, of course, the likeliest explanation. The pattern of the epidemic, the apparent absence of any common exposure factors, and the high incidence of illness among medical and hospital personnel were consistent only with an infectious disease transmitted from person to person. Just how the micro-organism responsible might travel from one person to another was not at all clear. It is still wide open to conjecture. We were able, however, to postulate the general nature of the micro-organism. It was probably a virus. It almost certainly wasn't one of the rickettsia. We did laboratory studies for all known rickettsial agents, and they were negative. Besides, the symptoms were wrong — most rickettsial diseases are characterized by high fever and a rash. Moreover, most of them are insect-borne. And it probably wasn't a bacterium. The laboratory studies were uniformly negative. It's true that they were negative for viruses as well as for bacteria, but the techniques for detecting bacteria are far better than those for detecting viruses. There is, of course, the possibility that the infection in epidemic neuro-myasthenia may occur quite early on and that by the time the patient sees a doctor he has stopped excreting the organism. That's not unheard of, you know. It happens in several virus diseases. And rheumatic fever follows a precipitating strepto-coccal infection by as much as a month. So does acute glom-erulonephritis. Nevertheless, if bacteria were involved, the chances are that we would have got something growing in the laboratory. Some hint of something would have sooner or later shown up. But not with a virus. The viruses are different. It's hard enough to find them in the best of circumstances. There are virus diseases in which no detectable change occurs in the white-blood-cell count, and they're extremely hard to culti-vate. They're extremely numerous, too. Umpteen new ones are discovered every year.

"There was a certain satisfaction in forming that hypothesis. It's nice to come to even the most tentative conclusion. One gets a sense of accomplishment. But it wasn't much of a com-fort. I mean, it didn't really explain a thing. The case was still a mystery. As a matter of fact, it was more than that. It was eerie. There's something a bit unnerving about a new com-municable disease — a disease whose cause and means of transmission are essentially unknown. I'll never forget the end of that first visit to Punta Gorda. We were able to relax later on, but we didn't know about that yet. It was the only time I've ever felt uneasy after an investigation about going straight home to my wife. For all I knew, I might have been exposed to epidemic neuromyasthenia, and I was worried about passing it on to her. I actually considered stopping over somewhere for several days and waiting to see what happened. The reason I didn't was that the incubation period was also a total mystery. I didn't know how long it would be advisable to wait.

"And yet, by the end of the investigation — by the end of our third and final visit — we did have a real sense of satisfaction. We could truthfully say that we had accomplished something. Our work here at the CDC is with communicable disease. We want to know all we can about it. And now we had had the experience of studying an outbreak of a new and mysterious communicable disease in detail. Reading about a disease is hardly the same as actually working on it. There's obviously a world of difference. We still know painfully little about epidemic neuromyasthenia, but Punta Gorda gave us at least some sense of what it is and what it isn't. We'll know it the next time we see it. And we'll have some new approaches to employ. It is now perfectly clear that medical and hospital people are especially vulnerable to epidemic neuromyasthenia, so we'll concentrate on them. We'll get to them as early as possible, we'll keep them under the closest possible observation, and we'll recover every possible specimen for laboratory study. In other words, we're ready and waiting. But Punta Gorda happened quite a few years ago, and I must say I'm beginning to wonder. I wonder if there will ever be a next time. The last reported outbreaks of epidemic neuromyasthenia occurred in 1958 in Athens, and in a convent up in New York State in 1961. Neither of them was recognized for what it was until it had almost run its course. We haven't heard even a decent rumor of it since then. It seems to have disappeared."

# The Huckleby Hogs

The telephone rang, and Dr. Likosky — William H.
Likosky, an Epidemic Intelligence Service officer attached to
the Neurotropic Viral Diseases Activity of the Center for
Disease Control, in Atlanta — reached across his desk and answered it, and heard the voice of a friend and fellow-EIS
officer named Paul Edward Pierce. Dr. Pierce was attached to
the New Mexico Department of Health and Social Services,
and he was calling from his office in Santa Fe. His call was a
call for help. Three cases of unusual illness had just been reported to him by a district health officer. The victims were
two girls and a boy, members of a family of nine, and they
lived in Alamogordo, a town of around twenty thousand, just
north of El Paso, Texas. The report noted that the family
raised hogs, and that several months earlier some of the hogs

had become sick and died. The children were seriously ill. Their symptoms included decreased vision, difficulty in walking, bizarre behavior, apathy, and coma. This complex of central-nervous-system aberrations had immediately suggested a viral encephalitis, but that, on reflection, seemed hardly possible. The encephalitides that he had in mind were spread by ticks or mosquitoes, and the season was wrong for insects. This was winter. It was, in fact, midwinter. It was January — January 7, 1970.

"I'm afraid I wasn't much help," Dr. Likosky says. "I could only listen and agree. It was just as Ed Pierce said. The clinical picture was characteristic of the kind of brain inflammation that distinguishes the viral encephalitides. More or less. But there were certainly some confusing elements. It wasn't only that the time of year was odd for arthropod-borne disease. The attack rate was odd, too. There were too many cases. A cluster like that is unusual in an arbovirus disease. Also, the report to Ed had made no mention of fever. That was odd in a serious virus infection. It was odd, but not necessarily conclusive. The report was just a preliminary report. It was very possibly incomplete. At any rate, Ed was driving down to Alamogordo the following day and he would see for himself. Things might look different on the scene. Meanwhile, about all I could suggest was the obvious. Verify the facts. Check into the possibility of a wintering mosquito population. Check up on the hogs. This might be a zoonosis — an animal disease. It might be a disease of hogs that the three children had somehow contracted. Review the signs and symptoms. Not only for fever but also for stiff neck. Stiff neck is particularly characteristic of encephalitis.

"That was a Wednesday. Ed called me from Alamogordo on

Friday. He and one of his colleagues — Jon Thompson, supervisor of the Food Protection Unit of the Consumer Protection Section of the state health department — had been out to the house, and he had some more information. The victims were children of a couple named Huckleby. They were Ernestine, eight years old; Amos Charles, thirteen; and Dorothy, eighteen. Ernestine was in the hospital — Providence Memorial Hospital, in El Paso. She had been there since just after Christmas. Amos Charles and Dorothy were sick at home. None of the other children — two girls and two boys — was sick, and neither were the parents. Huckleby worked as a janitor at a junior high school in Alamogordo. He only raised hogs on the side. All that was by way of background. The interesting information was about the Huckleby hogs. There were several items. The hog sickness happened back in October. Huckleby had a herd of seventeen hogs at the time, and all of a sudden one day fourteen of them were stricken with a sort of blind staggers — a stumbling gait and blindness. Twelve of the sick hogs died, and the two others went blind. That was interesting enough, but it was really only the beginning. In the course of their talk with Huckleby, Ed and Jon Thompson learned that the feed he gave his hogs included surplus seed grain. Well, seed grain isn't feed. Seed grain is chemically treated to resist all manner of diseases, and when it is past its season and loses its germination value, it is considered waste and is supposed to be destroyed. Huckleby said that the grain — it was a mixture of several grains, apparently — was the floor sweepings of a seed company upstate. He said a friend had given it to him, and he knew it contained treated grain. Or, rather, he knew it included treated grain. It was also partly chaff and culls. But he took care of that by cooking it with water and garbage in a metal trough before he fed it to his hogs. He said he had been given about two tons of the grain, and he still had some left. He also said that he had slaughtered one of his hogs back in September for home use. They had been eating it right along, but there was still some left in his freezer. Ed told him to leave it right where it was. There might be nothing wrong with it, but there was no use taking chances.

"Poison was a tempting possibility. The symptoms had the look of poison, but it wasn't a look that any of us were familiar with. That was the trouble. Nothing seemed to fit. Huckleby was even a little vague about whether the slaughtered hog had been fed the seed-grain feed. Moreover, he wasn't the only Alamogordan to feed that grain to his hogs. He said that five of his friends had got the same grain from the seed company, and none of their hogs had become ill. Apparently, that was true. Ed and Jon had talked with the other hog raisers. They weren't quite sure about the grain they had used, but they were positive that none of their hogs had sickened or died. The local records confirmed what they said. The local records also confirmed that the human outbreak was confined to the Huckleby family. There were no comparable illnesses any-where in the Alamogordo area. Ed and John had visited the butcher shop where the Huckleby hog had been processed. The butcher testified that the meat had appeared to be in prime condition. An examination of the shop was negative — there was nothing to suggest that the meat might have become contaminated during processing. And, finally, there was the fact that others in the family had eaten quantities of the pork, and only those three were sick. Nevertheless, Ed was taking the usual steps. He had samples of grain from Huckleby's storehouse, samples of pork from the family freezer, and samples of urine from all members of the family then at home — that is to say, all but Ernestine. He had arranged for the State Laboratory to examine those for viral or bacterial contamination, and he was sending specimens to William Barthel, chief of the Toxicology Branch Laboratory of the Food and Drug Administration, in Atlanta, for toxicological analysis. But even that wasn't all. Ed had still another piece of information. The clinical picture was pretty much as originally reported. Except in one respect. Ernestine's symptoms *did* include fever. High fever. A local doctor reported that her temperature at one point got up to 104 degrees. And — oh, yes, there were no mosquitoes in Alamogordo in January.

"I talked to Ed again on Saturday. He was back in Santa Fe, and that was the reason for his call. He called to invite me to participate in the field investigation. Ed had a big rubella-immunization program coming up at a Navajo reservation the next week that he couldn't put off, and there was nobody to run it but him. It was up to him to at least get it started. He had talked to his chief in New Mexico, Dr. Bruce Storrs, director of the Medical Services Division of the state health department, and he had talked to my boss at CDC, Dr. Michael Gregg, chief of the Viral Diseases Branch. They both approved the proposal. So did I. I was very eager."

Dr. Likosky left Atlanta by plane the following morning. That was Sunday, January 11. He flew to Albuquerque, where, by prearrangement, he met Dr. Pierce in the early evening. They talked and ate dinner and talked until nearly eleven. Dr. Likosky then rented a car and drove down through the mountains and the desert to Alamogordo. He spent the night (on Dr. Pierce's recommendation) at the Rocket Motel there, and on Monday morning (following Dr. Pierce's directions) he drove out to the Huckleby house.

"I wasn't checking up on Ed or Jon Thompson or the district health officer, or anything like that," Dr. Likosky says. "I simply wanted to see for myself. I wanted to start at the beginning. I got to the Huckleby house at about eight-thirty. Huckleby was at work, at the school, but Mrs. Huckleby was at home, and she received me very nicely. The first thing I learned was that Amos Charles and Dorothy were now also in Providence Memorial Hospital. They were too far gone in coma to be treated at home anymore. They had been taken down to El Paso only the day before. I liked Mrs. Huckleby at once. You could tell she was a good mother. Easygoing, but kind and loving. And she was going to be a mother once again. She was very obviously pregnant. The baby was due, she said, sometime in March. She was a religious woman, too, and that gave her a certain serenity. She believed that everything was in the hands of God. She was also an excellent historian. She remembered every detail of each child's illness. We began with Ernestine. She came home sick from school a little before noon on December 4. She said she had fallen off the monkey bars at recess, and she had a pain in her left lower back. Mrs. Huckleby said she felt hot to the touch. A few days went by, and Ernestine continued to complain of pain and just not feeling right. On December 8, Mrs. Huckleby took her to a neighborhood doctor. It was he who found that she had a temperature of 104, but he found nothing else of any significance. He prescribed aspirin and rest in bed. There was still no improvement, and on December 11 Mrs. Huckleby took her back to the doctor. It was a different doctor this time — the first doctor was off that day — and he did find something. He noticed that Ernestine wasn't walking right — that she was staggering — and he arranged to have her admitted to Providence Memorial the next day for observation. I got the details later from the doctor. Ernestine's walk and the history of her fall had frightened him a little. It raised the possibility in his mind of a subdural hematoma. A subdural hematoma is a gathering of blood between certain membranes that cover the brain. It is usually caused by a blow or a fall, and it can be extremely dangerous. I saw his point. It was a perfectly reasonable suspicion. But, of course, he was mistaken. It wasn't that. The hospital made the various tests, and ruled it out.

"Mrs. Huckleby told me that the hospital sent Ernestine home for Christmas. She was discharged on December 19. She got steadily worse during her stay at home, and she was readmitted on December 27. It was a pretty dreary Christmas for the Hucklebys. Amos Charles took sick while Ernestine was home — on Christmas Eve. He went to bed with an earache, and when he woke up Christmas morning, he said he couldn't see very well. The next day, Dorothy took sick. It began as a generalized malaise. Then she began to feel 'woobly.' Then she couldn't walk at all, and her speech began to slur. Meanwhile, much the same thing was happening to Amos Charles — trouble walking, trouble talking, trouble seeing. Then he went into what Mrs. Huckleby called a 'rage.' It was a good descriptive word. He was wild, uncoordinated, thrashing around on the bed. He and Dorothy both got steadily worse. They sank into coma. And, finally, on Sunday, they had to go into the hospital. I spent the rest of Monday talking to the Alamogordo doctors, and then to Huckleby. He wasn't easy to talk to. He was shy, and he didn't say much. He raised his hogs in a couple of pens he rented at a hog farm on the outskirts of town. He collected garbage from his neighbors, and he fed his hogs a mixture of that and grain and water. He cooked it because the law required that garbage be treated that way for feed. He stored his grain in a shed at home, and he kept the shed locked. I saw the grain — what was left of it. It was a mixture of grain and chaff. Anyone would have wondered about it. Most of the grain was coated with a pink warning dye. Huckleby said he had stopped feeding the grain as soon as he heard it was dangerous. I said I certainly hoped so. I questioned him particularly about the sickness that had afflicted his hogs in October. He told me this. When he saw his hogs one morning, they were well. When he saw them next, around four o'clock that afternoon, they were blind and staggering, sick and dying. That was strange. I hadn't ruled out encephalitis in the children, but this was different. There almost had to be a connection between the sick hogs and that chemically treated grain. And I couldn't connect a sudden illness and sudden death with any chronic poisoning.

"Everybody was still thinking in terms of encephalitis. That was the admitting diagnosis on Amos Charles and Dorothy at Providence Memorial Hospital. I spent Tuesday and Wednesday in El Paso. I read the records and I talked to the doctors involved. The relevant test results were either normal or not very helpful. The children's kind of blindness was identified as tunnel, or gun-barrel, vision — a constriction of the visual fields. Urinalysis was positive for protein in all three patients, and the presence of protein in the urine always indicates some impairment of function, which is unusual in most encephalitides. And I saw the patients. It was terrible. I'll never forget them. It was shattering. Amos Charles was a big, husky, good-looking boy, and he lay there just a vegetable. His brain was gone. Ernestine was much the same. Dorothy was a little more alive. Her arms kept waving back and forth. Pendular ataxia, it's called. The charts on the children spelled everything out.

"I talked to Ed on Tuesday afternoon, and he drove down to El Paso that night. He had his rubella campaign well started, and he was eager to get back into the Huckleby investigation. He brought some confusing news along. One of Jon Thompson's people had run down the source of Huckleby's grain and identified at least one formulation of the material it was treated with. It was a fungicide called Panogen. Panogen is cyano methyl mercury guanidine. And mercury is a classic poison. It's one of the most dangerous of the heavy metals. Well, that should have clarified things a bit, but it didn't. It only added to the confusion. Because the clinical picture the Huckleby children presented looked nothing like classic mercury poisoning. The textbook symptoms of acute mercury poisoning are essentially gastrointestinal — nausea, vomiting, abdominal pain, bloody stools. That and severe kidney damage. Chronic mercury poisoning is entirely different. The kidneys are not seriously involved. Apparently, they can safely handle small amounts of mercury. The features in chronic mercurialism are an inflammation of the mouth, muscular tremors — the famous hatter's shakes — and a characteristic personality change. Shyness, embarrassment, irritability. Like the Mad Hatter in *Alice in Wonderland*. We didn't know what to think.

"We couldn't dismiss the possibility of mercury. But we couldn't quite accept it, either. The only thing we were finally certain about was that we weren't up against an acute viral encephalitis. The clinical picture — particularly the gradual development of symptoms — and the epidemiology made it quite unlikely. It made it incredible. We decided that we were left with two general possibilities. One was a more insidious kind of encephalitis — a slow-moving viral infection of the brain. The other was an encephalopathy. Encephalitis is a disease of the gray matter — or gray nervous tissue — of the brain. Encephalopathy involves the white matter — the conducting nerve fibres. A toxic encephalopathy was the kind we chiefly had in mind. The cause could be one of a variety of substances. The heavy metals, of course. Arsenic. Or numerous drugs on the order of sedatives and tranquilizers. The slow-moving-viral possibilities were more exotic. Rabies is in that class. And kuru, a fatal neurological infection in New Guinea that is perpetuated by cannibalism. And scrapie, a disease of sheep, but a human possibility. And others. The trouble was that Ed and I weren't neurologists. But I had a friend who was — Dr. James Schwartz, at Emory University, in Atlanta. So, just on a chance, I called him up and gave him the clinical picture and asked him what *he* thought it sounded like. He gave us quite a shock. He said it sounded a lot like one of the multiple scleroses — a rapidly progressive demyelinating process called Schilder's disease. Except, he said, three cases would constitute an epidemic, and an epidemic of Schilder's disease had never been reported before. He was inclined to doubt that one ever would be. Another, and more reasonable, possibility, he said, was heavy-metal poisoning. Except that our picture wasn't quite right for lead. Or mercury. Or anything else that readily came to mind. I thanked him just the same. Ed and I decided we had better go back to Alamogordo.

"We went back on Thursday. Jon Thompson joined us there, and we spent most of the day at the Huckleby house, taking it apart. It would have been very exciting to turn up the first epidemic of Schilder's disease in history, but we decided that my talk with Dr. Schwartz had just about narrowed the possibilities down to a toxic encephalopathy, and we were looking for a possible source of poisoning. Ed and Jon had already searched the house, of course, but this time we really left no stone unturned. We went through every room and everything in every room. We went through the medicine cabinet. We checked the cooking utensils. Some pottery clay, for example, is mixed with lead, and there is sometimes lead in old pots and pans. We looked for spoiled food. We examined everything in the family freezer, including what was left of the hog they slaughtered back in September. We didn't find anything new or suspicious, though. We had another useless talk with Huckleby, and ate dinner and went back to the motel, and we were sitting there around eleven o'clock trying to think of what to do next — when the telephone rang. It was a call for me from Dr. Alan Hinman, in Atlanta. Alan was one of my bosses. He's the assistant chief to Mike Gregg in the Viral Diseases Branch at CDC, and he was calling from his office — at one o'clock in the morning! It was fantastic. And then it got more fantastic.

"Here's what Alan had to tell me. That afternoon, he said, just before quitting time, Mike Gregg had gone in to see Alexander Langmuir — Dr. Langmuir was then director of the Epidemiology Program at CDC — about something, and as he was leaving, he mentioned the Huckleby outbreak. Mike said there was this damn disease out in New Mexico with gunbarrel vision and ataxia and coma, and we didn't know what to make of it. Dr. Langmuir said oh? Then he stopped and blinked, and said it sounded to him as if it might be Minamata disease. Mike looked blank. Dr. Langmuir laughed, and picked up a reprint on his desk. He said his secretary had dumped a pile of accumulated reprints on his desk to either discard or keep on file, and this was one he had just finished looking at. It was a paper from *World Neurology* for November 1960, and it was entitled 'Minamata Disease: The Outbreak of a Neurologic Disorder in Minamata, Japan, and Its Relationship to the Ingestion of Seafood Contaminated by Mercuric Compounds.' Well, Mike took it home and read it, and it struck him just as hard. So he called up Alan, and Alan came over and got the reprint and read it, and he reacted in the same way, only more so. He drove down to the office and got into the library and checked the references, and there wasn't any question in his mind. Our problem was Minamata disease. He read me the original paper. It began like this: 'In 1958, a severe neurologic disorder was first recognized among persons living in the vicinity of Minamata Bay, Japan. Now 83 cases have been recorded, most ending fatally or with permanent severe disability. Epidemiologic investigations . . . helped to establish the relationship of this illness to the consumption of seafood from Minamata Bay. The effluent from a large chemical manufacturing plant which emptied into the bay had been suspected as the source of a toxic material contaminating fish and shellfish. Subsequent work has provided evidence that the responsible toxin is associated with the discharge of organic-mercury-containing effluent from the chemical factory.' The clinical features had a familiar sound. Ataxic gait. Clumsiness of the hands. Dysarthria, or slurred speech. Dysphagia, or difficulty in swallowing. Constriction of the visual fields. Deafness. Spasticity. Agitation. Stupor and coma. And this: 'Intellectual impairment occurs in severely affected patients; children seem particularly liable to serious residual defects.' And, finally, there was this: 'When the first cases were recognized, Japanese B encephalitis was considered as a diagnostic possibility; however, evidence against encephalitis (aside from the cardinal clinical features) includes the following: the onset of symptoms was usually subacute and not accompanied by fever, cases were limited geographically, and they occurred throughout the year.' The Minamata paper would have been enough for me, but Alan had found another that was even more convincing. It had the title 'Epidemiological Study of an Illness in the Guatemala Highlands Believed to Be Encephalitis,' and it had been published in the *Boletín de la Oficina Sanitaria Panamericana* in 1966. The passage that really clinched it was this: 'Possible toxic elements in food, such as edible mushrooms, were investigated. In the course of this investigation it was noted that during the period of the year in which the illness occurred, many families, and especially the poorest, ate part of the wheat given them for seed, which had been treated with a fungicide known commercially as Panogen — an organic-mercury compound.'

"That was the key — that word 'organic.' It instantly clarified everything. Panogen is cyano methyl mercury guanidine, and cyano methyl mercury guanidine is an *organic* mercury compound. Ed and I were perfectly well aware of that, but the significance just hadn't penetrated. When we thought of mercury, we naturally thought of *inorganic* mercury. That's the usual source of mercurialism. But the pathology of the two afflictions is very different. *Organic*-mercury poisoning has always been something of a rarity. Until recently, anyway. At the time of the Minamata report, the total number of cases of organic mercurialism on record was only thirty-nine. And only five of them were American. Well, I finally finished talking to Alan and gave the news to Ed and Jon, and we all immediately agreed. It was a fantastic kind of coincidence — Dr. Langmuir, Minamata, Guatemala. But it fitted to the letter. Or practically. Talking it over, we did see one objection. The behavior of the Huckleby hogs. Chronic poisoning doesn't produce a sudden, fatal illness. It doesn't, and — the way it turned out — it didn't. On Monday, January 19, I went out and had another talk with Huckleby, and I don't know why, but this time we got along much better than we had before, and he finally said that he could have been mistaken — that it probably wasn't all that sudden, that his hogs probably did get sicker and sicker over a period of several weeks.

"The only thing we needed now was proof. It arrived that night — Monday night — in another call from Alan. He had had a call from Mr. Barthel at the Toxicology Laboratory. Mr. Barthel had analyzed Ed's samples of grain and pork and urine, and he had found mercury in everything but two of the urine samples. The two negative samples were those of the two youngest Huckleby children. One of them was two years old and the other was just ten months, and neither of them had eaten any of the pork. The highest mercury levels were found in the patients' urine. That, of course, was as expected. One of the lowest was Mrs. Huckleby's. Which was fortunate. After all, she was pregnant. But the fact that she and the other asymptomatic members of the family showed any mercury at all was unexpected. It raised a question, and it was a question that would have bothered us if we hadn't been doing a little reading in the literature on our own. The question was: Why didn't *all* the pork-eating Hucklebys get sick? They all consumed about the same amount of meat. We found an acceptable answer in a 1940 paper in the British *Quarterly Journal of Medicine*. The paper was entitled 'Poisoning by Methyl Mercury Compounds,' and the relevant passage read, 'The fact that eight men, exposed in a similar way to the four patients, excreted mercury in the urine, yet showed no symptoms or signs of disease, suggests that most of the workers absorbed mercury compounds, but that only four . . . were susceptible to them.' That was the best explanation — Ernestine and Amos Charles and Dorothy were simply more susceptible to mercury than the others. It satisfied me, anyway. And the next day I flew home to Atlanta."

The chain of laboratory evidence that linked the Huckleby children's affliction to the diet of the Huckleby hogs brought the epidemiological investigation of the outbreak to an end. As it happened, however, that was not the end of the case. On Monday, January 19 — the day on which Dr. Likosky and Dr. Pierce and Mr. Thompson wound up their joint investigation — the case took a new and ominous turn.

The turn occurred in Clovis, New Mexico, a livestock center some two hundred miles northeast of Alamogordo, and it was set in motion by a state sanitarian on duty there named Cade Lancaster. Mr. Lancaster was the investigator who had identified Panogen as a chemical contaminant in the Huckleby grain. His second contribution to the case stemmed from a monitoring impulse that prompted him to leaf through the recent records of a Clovis hog broker. He didn't have far to look — only back to Friday, January 16. On that day, he was interested to read, the broker had bought a consignment of twenty-four hogs from a grower in Alamogordo. What particularly interested Mr. Lancaster was the grower's name. He knew it: the man was one of the Huckleby group who had included treated grain in their hog feed. He also knew that all the growers in that group had been instructed to withhold their hogs from market until otherwise notified. The feeding of treated grain had been stopped by horrified common consent at the very start of the investigation, but that was not enough to render the hogs safe for immediate use. Organic mercury is eliminated slowly from living tissue. It has a half-life there of two or three months. Mr. Lancaster sought out the broker. The broker stood appalled. He hadn't known. He had had no way of knowing. What was worse, he added, he had already disposed of the hogs. They were part of a shipment of two hundred forty-eight hogs that had gone out on Friday afternoon to a packing plant in Roswell. Mr. Lancaster turned to the telephone.

The recipient of Mr. Lancaster's call was Carl Henderson, chief of the Consumer Protection Section of the New Mexico Health and Social Services Department, and he received it in his office at Santa Fe. He thanked Mr. Lancaster for his enterprise, and sat in thought for a moment. Then he himself put in a call — to the packing plant in Roswell. The manager there heard the news with a groan. Yes, he said, he had the Alamo-gordo hogs, but that was the most he could say. He didn't know which they were. They were no longer hogs. The big Clovis shipment had been slaughtered on Saturday, and it was simply so many carcasses now. In that case, Mr. Henderson said, he had no choice but to immobilize the lot. The plant was therewith informed that all those two hundred forty-eight carcasses were under state embargo. Mr. Henderson hung up and moved to reinforce his pronouncement. His move was at once effective. The following day, January 20, the United States Department of Agriculture, through the Slaughter Inspection Division of its Consumer and Marketing Service, placed the state-embargoed carcasses under the further and stronger restraint of a federal embargo, and arranged for a sample of each carcass to be tested for mercury at the Agricultural Research Center, in Beltsville, Maryland. That same day, the state extended its embargo to the grain-fed hogs still in the possession of Huckleby and his five companion growers in Alamogordo. The next day, the hogs were tallied and found to total two hundred and fifteen head. One hog was selected from each grower's herd and killed and autopsied, and specimens were sent to the Toxicology Laboratory of the Food and Drug Administration, in Atlanta, for definitive examination.

Two days later, still shaken by Mr. Lancaster's discovery, the New Mexico Health and Social Services Department took another protective step. A cautionary letter, signed by Dr. Bruce D. Storrs, director of the Medical Services Division, was distributed to every physician and veterinarian in the state. The letter read:

A recent outbreak of central-nervous-system disease among three children of an Alamogordo family has been traced to the ingestion of pork contaminated with a methyl-mercury compound. The animal involved had been fed over a period of several weeks with grain treated with this material. At the time it was butchered, the hog appeared to be in good health, and visual inspection of the carcass during processing failed to reveal any significant abnormalities. Laboratory analysis of the meat eaten by the family, however, revealed a high concentration of methyl mercury.

The grain had been obtained by the children's father, free of charge, in the form of castoff "sweepings" from a seed company located in eastern New Mexico. This was mixed with garbage and fed to the hogs despite the knowledge that it had been treated with the fungicide. Several weeks after slaughter of the boar, 14 of the family's remaining 17 hogs became ill with symptoms of blindness and staggering gait. Over a three-week period, 12 died and the remaining two were permanently blind.

Because of the potential danger to humans of ingesting meat contaminated with methyl mercury (all three children are comatose and in critical condition), as well as the likelihood that the practice of feeding treated grain may be widespread among indigents raising livestock in the state, this matter is being brought to your attention. The possibility of methyl-mercury poisoning should be considered in any outbreak of . . . unusual central-nervous-system illness. Please notify the Preventive Medicine Section (Phone 505-827-2475) of any such occurrence, and we in turn will be happy to provide technical advice and assistance.

The letters were mailed out on Thursday, January 22. The Preventive Medicine Section spent Friday and the weekend waiting for the ring of the telephone and the urgent voice of a doctor. But nothing happened. Nothing happened the following week. February loomed, and began. Still nothing. The Preventive Medicine Section sat back and relaxed. They let themselves assume — correctly, as it turned out — that the outbreak was confined to the Huckleby family.

Nevertheless — as it also turned out — the danger of an epidemic had been real. Early in February, the results of the hog examinations were announced. The first report was on the embargoed packing-plant carcasses. It seemed to justify Mr. Lancaster's investigatory zeal, but its meaning was otherwise not entirely clear. Of the two hundred forty-eight carcasses examined by the Department of Agriculture, one — just one — was found to contain a high concentration of mercury. The others, curiously, were uncontaminated. The contaminated carcass was ordered destroyed, and the others were released to the market. The Toxicology Laboratory's report on the hogs taken from the Alamogordo pens was very different. Six hogs were examined, and all six were found to be dangerously contaminated with mercury. This unequivocal finding condemned the remaining hogs in the pens, and the state issued an order for their destruction.

Dr. Likosky returned to Atlanta with the Huckleby outbreak still very much on his mind. What particularly disturbed him was its implications. This led him back to the library, and he undertook a comprehensive exploration of the literature on organic mercury compounds and organic mercurialism. It was not a reassuring experience. Mercury fungicides, he learned, were developed in Germany around 1914 and came into almost universal use shortly after the First World War. He learned that the Minamata episode was not the only outbreak of organic-mercury poisoning caused by contaminated fish. It was merely the first. In 1965, despite the morbid Minamata example, a similar outbreak occurred on the Japanese island of Honshu. A total of a hundred twenty people were stricken there, and five of them died. He learned that the Guatemalan episode was not the only instance on record of poisoning caused by eating treated grain. A similar outbreak occurred in Iraq in 1961, and another in Pakistan in 1963. A total of almost five hundred people were struck down in the three outbreaks, and the mortality rate was high. He learned that the Huckleby hogs were not the first American hogs to be stricken with chronic mercury poisoning. They were merely the first involved in human mercurialism. He learned that Sweden had, on February 1, 1966, revoked the license for the use of certain highly toxic mercury compounds (including methyl mercury) in agriculture. He learned that the 1969 pheasant-hunting season in the Canadian province of Alberta had been canceled after a survey of the pheasant population showed an average mercury level of one part per million — a hazardous concentration. And, closer to home, he learned that a similar survey in Montana that same year revealed a level of mercury contamination that prompted the State Game Commission to advise hunters against eating the birds they shot. In both instances, the pheasants had been exposed in the field to treated seed.

Dr. Likosky arose from his reading with a sense of apprehension. He sought out two of his colleagues, Dr. Hinman and Mr. Barthel, chief of the Toxicology Branch, and found that they shared his concern about the proliferating casual use of a substance as toxic as methyl mercury. They also felt that a broader discussion of the matter was desirable, and Mr. Barthel arranged for a meeting in Washington with interested representatives of the Department of Agriculture and of the Food and Drug Administration. At the meeting, which was held on February 12, Dr. Likosky, Dr. Hinman, and Mr. Barthel reviewed the Huckleby case and its varied antecedents, and suggested that they constituted a looming public-health problem. Their arguments were well received, and on February 19 the Department of Agriculture issued a statement on the subject. It read:

The U.S. Department of Agriculture has notified pesticide manufacturers that Federal registrations are suspended for products containing cyano methyl mercury guanidine that are labeled for use as seed treatments.

U.S.D.A.'s Agricultural Research Service suspended cyano methyl mercury guanidine fungicide because its continued use on seeds would constitute an imminent hazard to the public health. Directions for proper use and caution statements on labels of the product have failed to prevent its misuse as a livestock feed. The U.S.D.A.-registered label specifically warns against use of mercury-treated seed for food or feed purposes. The pesticide may cause irreversible damage to both animals and man.

The action was taken following the hospitalization of three New

Mexico children after they ate meat from a hog which had been fed seed grain treated with the now-suspended mercury compound. Subsequently, 12 of the remaining 14 hogs also fed the seed died.

"Other movements of this treated seed that found its way into livestock feed posed a potential for similar incidents," Dr. Harry W. Hays, director of the Pesticides Regulations Division, USDA-ARS, said in announcing the suspension action. "In each case, USDA and state public health officials have taken prompt action to protect the public health." Dr. Hays also announced that the ARS had asked the Advisory Center on Toxicology of the National Research Council to review the uses of other organic-mercury compounds to determine whether similar hazards to human health existed in connection with the use of these compounds.

March came on. Ernestine and Amos Charles Huckleby were discharged from Providence Memorial Hospital, in El Paso, and transferred to the chronic-care facility of a hospital in Alamogordo. They were still comatose. (Ernestine will probably be permanently comatose. She is almost certainly blind. Amos can communicate on a primitive level. He, too, is blind.) At the same time, Dorothy Huckleby was removed to a rehabilitation hospital in Roswell. (It is expected that she may in time recover enough to care for herself under general supervision.) Meanwhile, Mrs. Huckleby's term approached. Because of the delicate nature of her pregnancy, state health officials had recommended that her confinement take place in the scientifically sophisticated environment of the University of New Mexico Medical Center, in Albuquerque, and she was admitted to a maternity ward there. Her condition was satisfactory and her course was uneventful. On Monday, March 9, she was delivered of a seven-pound boy. At birth, the baby appeared to be physically normal, but a few hours later he experienced a violent convulsion. He survived the seizure, and recovered. The prognosis, however, was uncertain. It is very possible, in view of his long fetal exposure to mercury, that some physical or mental abnormalities will eventually manifest themselves.

April arrived. Manufacturers affected by the federal suspension order on seed dressings containing cyano methyl mercury guanidine stirred, and suddenly struck. On April 10, Morton International, Inc., and its subsidiary Nor-Am Agricultural Products, Inc., the makers of Panogen, applied in United States District Court in Chicago for an injunction relieving the company of compliance with the suspension order, and the application was granted by Judge Alexander J. Napoli. The grounds for granting the injunction were that the Department of Agriculture had acted without holding a hearing to establish the hazardous nature of the fungicide.

The government appealed, and on July 15 a three-judge panel of the Court of Appeals turned the government down, again citing insufficient evidence. The government then petitioned for a review by all six judges of the Court of Appeals. This request was granted, and the full panel met and reviewed the case. Their decision was announced on November 9. The panel ruled, by a vote of four to two, to uphold the government suspension. Thus, after almost seven months of swinging in the wind of legal technicalities, the door was closed again on methyl mercury guanidine dressings, and this time firmly latched.

# The Hiccups

Among the several patients who consulted Dr. Heinz B. Eisenstadt, an internist, at his office in Port Arthur, Texas, on the morning of February 13, 1945, was a sixty-year-old oil-refinery worker whom I'll call Eliot Warren. Warren's appointment identified him as a new patient, and, as was usual in such cases, his medical history was recorded by a nurse in a cubicle off the reception room. It showed that he had undergone a hernia operation in 1940, and that he suffered from hives (after eating certain foods), hay fever (in season), asthma, and a frequent need to urinate. This visit, however, had nothing to do with any of those afflictions. His present complaint, he told the nurse, was what he took to be an attack of indigestion. He had been troubled for almost a week with flatulence and heartburn. Dr. Eisenstadt had the nurse's report on his desk when Warren was shown into his office. He could see no cause for serious concern in either Warren's past or present problems, and an immediate freehand examination confirmed that first impression. Warren's allergic susceptibilities were essentially unimportant, his asthmatic symptoms were a manifestation of a mild emphysema, his urinary difficulties were the natural consequence of a moderate (and, in a man of sixty, more or less normal) enlargement of the prostate gland, and his indigestion was probably simple indigestion. Dr. Eisenstadt explained these observations to Warren, and then turned him over to a technician for a definitive appraisal — a chest X-ray, an electrocardiogram, and the standard laboratory tests. Such an appraisal, he said, was merely prudent. He was confident that Warren had nothing to worry about. Meanwhile, he added, he would draw up a prescription to ease his stomach and a diet to keep it easy.

Dr. Eisenstadt didn't expect to see Warren soon again, and he didn't. Warren had not been a memorable patient, and Dr. Eisenstadt almost at once forgot him. Warren remained forgotten for almost exactly four years — until March 1, 1949. On the morning of that day, he reappeared at Dr. Eisenstadt's office with what sounded like the same complaint as before. Also, he had the hiccups. He had been hiccuping off and on for several weeks. Some of the spells had lasted as long as two or three hours, and he was beginning to get worried. He had tried all the home remedies that were known in his home, but none of them had worked. When the hiccups stopped, they simply stopped. Warren added that he had had a similar experience back in 1940. That was the year of his hernia operation, and, as well as he could remember, the hiccups had happened around that time. Dr. Eisenstadt made a perfunctory note. He couldn't see any real connection between that experience of hiccups and this. He could, however, see one between these spells and the chronic indigestion about which Warren had consulted him in 1945. Indigestion — gastric irritation — is the usual cause of hiccups. But his first concern was for Warren's comfort. He wrote out a prescription for what he hoped would be a curative combination of codeine, phenobarbital, and belladonna. He then reviewed Warren's diet. That seemed to confirm the cause of the trouble: Warren had drifted away from most of the 1945 recommendations. Dr. Eisenstadt put him firmly back on a proper bland regimen.

That was a Tuesday. Six days later, on Monday, March 7, Dr. Eisenstadt received a telephone call from Warren. The reason for the call was only too apparent. Warren had the hiccups. Dr. Eisenstadt told him to come at once to the office, and he was ready for him when he arrived. He gave him an intravenous injection of a respiratory and central-nervous-system stimulant called nikethamide. Nikethamide is a power-ful drug, and it had a powerful effect on Warren. He gave a gasp — an enormous gasp — and his hiccups stopped. The at-tack had lasted for five or six hours, and the relief he now felt was exquisite. It enabled him to think of other things — other problems. He reported to Dr. Eisenstadt that he still had trou-ble urinating. In fact, he thought, it was worse than before. Dr. Eisenstadt examined his prostate. Four years had made a difference. It was considerably enlarged. Dr. Eisenstadt gave him a prostatic massage, and that seemed to help. Warren left the office in good spirits.

Two weeks went by. Dr. Eisenstadt heard nothing more from Warren, and he found his silence gratifying. The nike-thamide injection had apparently had a lasting impact. But it hadn't. Warren's hiccups returned on the morning of March 24, and that afternoon he was back in Dr. Eisenstadt's office. Dr. Eisenstadt did as he had done before. He gave Warren an injection of nikethamide, and again the hiccups stopped. But this time they hardly stayed stopped at all. Warren was back again the next afternoon in the clutch of another seizure. Dr. Eisenstadt's confidence in nikethamide was shaken but not yet shattered. He gave Warren another injection, and it worked as it had before — exactly as before. It stopped the hiccups, but only for a matter of hours. They returned the following morning. Nevertheless, Dr. Eisenstadt tried nikethamide once again. He knew it would give Warren at least some relief, and he hoped it would do more than that. If it didn't, he decided, Warren would have to go into the hospital. He would need the kind of treatment that only a hospital can provide. The nikethamide failed to recover its enduring original power, and the hiccups were back the next morning. That was March 27. Dr. Eisenstadt called St. Mary's Hospital and made the necessary arrangements, and Warren was admitted there that afternoon for observation and treatment of persistent hiccups.

A hiccup (or, as medical pedants sometimes prefer, singultus) is the strangulating result of a spasmodic contraction of the diaphragm. It occurs when the massive intake of air thus involuntarily induced is abruptly checked by a sudden, arbitrary closure of the windpipe. The name of the phenomenon derives from the sound of that explosive interruption. In this onomatopoeic respect, the hiccup resembles the cough, the sneeze, and the belch, and it is also, like those similarly spontaneous spasms, a physiological commonplace. There, however, the similarity ceases. The cough, the sneeze, and the belch are all protective reactions. They are an essential part of the body's defensive apparatus: they clear the throat, they open the nose, they ease the bloated stomach. Hiccups serve no useful purpose. They are purely pathological. At best, they are merely innocuous. At worst, they can be, and often have been, fatal.

The immediate cause of the hiccup spasm is a reflex set in motion by an abnormal stimulation of the conductors that control the diaphragm and the opening (which science calls the glottis) at the mouth of the windpipe. These conductors are the phrenic and the vagus nerves. The stimulation that excites these nerves may be direct or it may have its origin in the central nervous system. Almost any disease, including (particularly in women) psychogenic disorders, thus has the power to precipitate an attack of hiccups, and, for the same reason, hiccups are a not uncommon aftermath of serious surgery. Hiccup spasms, being reflex actions, occur with metronomic regularity, but the tempo may be fast or slow. In dangerous attacks (those that persist for forty-eight hours or more), the beat is always fast. Persistent hiccups usually appear in tandem with some serious disease or condition. The severity of an attack of hiccups is determined by its duration, and it is persistence — hour after hour of jolting, jarring, breath-taking, sleepless spasms — that makes hiccups dangerous.

The treatment of hiccups involves the interruption of the perpetuating reflex. Once its regular rhythm is broken, the spasms generally cease. Simple hiccups — the hiccups that follow the bolted meal or the ultimate drink — respond to simple devices. There are many such devices, and most of them are very old. Some understanding of the cause and cure of simple hiccups is probably as old as the hiccups themselves. Plato, in the fourth century B.C., enlivened the Dialogue that he called the "Symposium" with a sudden attack of the hiccups: "The turn of Aristophanes was next, but either he had eaten too much, or from some other cause [he had been "drowned in drink" the day before], he had the hiccough." Aristophanes is advised by Eryximachus, "Let me recommend you to hold your breath, and if after you have done so for some time the hiccough is no better, then gargle with a little water; and if it still continues, tickle your nose with something and sneeze; and if you sneeze once or twice, even the most violent hiccough is sure to go." A few minutes later, Aristophanes announces, "The hiccough is gone. . . . I no sooner applied the sneezing than I was cured." Sneezing was the remedy most favored by Hippocrates. He seems, moreover, to have understood why it worked. "If sneezing is produced," he notes in the clinical testament known as *Aphorisms*, "the singultus being temporarily suppressed, the singultus will be cured." The first-century Roman encyclopedist Pliny also recommended sneezing. "To sneeze," he notes in his *Natural History*, "is a ready way to be rid of the yex or hiccough." Sneezing was one of several similarly effective remedies proposed by the eighteenth-century German physician Valentino Krauetermann. In a book called *Der Thueringische Theophrastus Paracelsus, Wunder-und Kraueterdoctor, oder der curieuse und verneunftige Zauber-Arzt*, he notes, "Some cure [the hiccups] by unexpectedly frightening the patient. Some say to rub the little finger in the ears; some hold the breath or sneeze." Other standard remedies long listed in the folk pharmacopoeia include a cold compress on the back of the neck, a glass or two of cold water drunk slowly, and a sharp pull on the tongue. All of these several remedies are empirical remedies. They were discovered by some happy accident, and they have survived because — though for reasons unknown to the discoverer (the phrenic nerve, for example, runs up the side of the neck) — they more or less consistently work. The most reliable of the empirical hiccup cures is a refinement of Eryximachus's first recommendation. It is also ingeniously simple. The patient, instead of holding his breath, merely breathes for two or three minutes into a paper bag. Breathing and rebreathing the air in the bag increases, first, the amount of carbon dioxide in the bag, then the carbon dioxide in the lungs, and, finally, the carbon dioxide in the blood. This emergency arouses the respiratory centers in the brain to defensive action. They move to eliminate the dangerous concentration of carbon dioxide by quickening and deepening the contractions of the diaphragm, and the hiccup spasms are tripped and broken.

The dyspeptical hiccup remedies have no effect on hiccups of more complicated origin. They are too feeble to interrupt the spasms that spring from powerful provocation. Persistent hiccups give way, if at all, only to overwhelming pressures. The most overwhelming of these maneuvers is surgical — one of the phrenic nerves (usually the left) is exposed and blocked. Another approach is chemical. This includes the administration of such variously potent drugs as anti-spasmodics, muscle relaxants, respiratory stimulants, and central-nervous-system depressants. A third approach is an absolute refinement of the paper-bag technique. The paper bag is here replaced by a machine that produces a mixture of five to ten percent carbon dioxide in oxygen. The patient, masked and closely attended, breathes that near-toxic air for several minutes (but no more than ten) every hour until his hiccups cease — or until he feels a warning wave of dizziness. It was to receive this often magisterial treatment that Eliot Warren was admitted to St. Mary's Hospital on the afternoon of March 27, 1949.

Warren spent a week at St. Mary's. The carbon-dioxide-inhalation treatment was at first only briefly effective, but then the intervals between attacks began to lengthen. They grew from hours to a day to days. By the seventh hospital day — on Saturday, April 2 — it was clear that the seizure was over, and Warren was discharged that afternoon. Dr. Eisenstadt saw him out with a comfortable combination of relief and satisfaction. He was relieved that Warren's hiccups had finally relented, and he was satisfied that he knew their probable cause. He didn't think it was indigestion again. These hiccups were too persistent for that. But the hospital had offered a clue. A series of diagnostic tests and examinations showed that Warren's general debilities now included an incipient cerebral arteriosclerosis. His arteries were beginning to harden. It was Dr. Eisenstadt's guess that Warren had recently suffered a little stroke. Little strokes — strokes so slight that they do no perceptible damage — are not uncommon in men past sixty. Warren's arteriosclerotic condition favored such a stroke, and such a stroke could easily have produced the neural excitation necessary to set off a prolonged attack of hiccups. Dr. Eisenstadt closed his record of the episode with that tentative explanation.

Warren faded once again from Dr. Eisenstadt's mind. He was recalled, but only for a moment, in the spring of 1951. Dr. Eisenstadt had been away on a short vacation. When he returned to his office, he found among the reports left by his locum tenens a note on a visit from Warren. Warren's complaint was hiccups — intermittent hiccups of three days' duration. The doctor had prescribed, apparently successfully, a sedative. Two more years went by. Then, on June 22, 1953, Warren turned up again. But it wasn't hiccups this time. The symptoms that prompted his visit were swollen ankles, shortness of breath, and a recent gain in weight. Dr. Eisenstadt's interpretation of these conspicuously dropsical signs was conventional. In view of Warren's arteriosclerotic history, they almost certainly pointed to congestive heart failure. At the moment, he thought, it was not an unduly dangerous condition, but he prescribed the conventional treatment: digitalis, once a day. He then asked Warren about his other, established complaints. Warren thought they were much the same. Two years ago, not long before his last visit, he had suffered a painful attack of prostatitis, and a urologist he consulted had performed an alleviative transurethral resection — but that was all. What about hiccups? Warren shook his head. He hadn't had a real hiccup in months. He thought they were gone for good.

Warren spoke a bit too soon. Three weeks later, on July 12, Dr. Eisenstadt got a telephone call from Warren's urologist. Warren was back in St. Mary's Hospital. His prostate was again inflamed, and he had been admitted the day before for a cystoscopic (or direct) examination to evaluate the nature of the trouble. The cystoscopy had been reassuring — no sign of any serious disease. But shortly after the operation Warren had begun to hiccup, and he had been hiccuping ever since. Would Dr. Eisenstadt, as Warren's family physician, come over and lend a hand? Dr. Eisenstadt would, and did. He treated Warren first with carbon dioxide, and then, when that failed to firmly subdue the spasms, with a respiratory stimulant called pentylenetetrazol. Pentylenetetrazol, after almost a week, brought the attack to an end. But what had caused this attack? Warren's general condition seemed much as usual. Dr. Eisenstadt was at a loss for several days. He finally decided to attribute the attack to the stress and strain of the cystoscopic examination.

Another interlude occurred. Warren came to Dr. Eisenstadt's attention just four times in the course of the next twelve years. He saw him once in 1955, once in 1958, and twice in 1962. Three were office calls, and one was a hospital visit. The 1955 consultation was for a sudden recurrence of the hiccups. It was not a vigorous attack, and Dr. Eisenstadt treated it successfully with a muscle relaxant called quinidine. The cause of the attack appeared to be a return of Warren's chronically recurrent indigestion. It was an attack of indigestion — including heartburn, nausea, and vomiting — that brought Warren into Dr. Eisenstadt's office in 1958. Dr. Eisenstadt satisfied himself that it was indeed an attack of indigestion, and then treated Warren with a soothing drug and another warning word on diet. He also took advantage of the occasion to give him a comprehensive checkup. This confirmed that Warren's several ailments were still progressing at an unhurried rate commensurate with his age. It also added a new debility to the list. Warren now had a mild and easily controllable diabetes mellitus. The first of the 1962 visits was brought about by another prostate operation — a transurethral re-resection. Dr. Eisenstadt's role was that of a clinical consultant to the urologist. He determined that Warren had the stamina to endure such an operation, and then stood by in case an attack of post-operative hiccups broke out. One did, but he brought it quickly to heel with Dramamine. The other 1962 visit occurred only two weeks later. It was a routine post-operative consultation, and Dr. Eisenstadt's findings were entirely routine.

Warren turned eighty in 1965. He was still active enough for his limited needs and notions, but the burden of ailments that he carried now was considerable. Dr. Eisenstadt examined him in February of that year and found that he was suffering from general arteriosclerosis, congestive heart failure, coronary heart disease, emphysema, chronic indigestion, prostatic hypertrophy, diabetes, hay fever, phlebitis (in the left leg), and gallstones. None, however, was alarmingly advanced, and most of them were held in tolerable check by drugs. The drugs that performed these services were also notably numerous. Dr. Eisenstadt ran down the list. It included digitalis, an aluminum hydroxide stomachic, a diuretic (to control the edema resulting from his congestive heart failure), an antihistamine (to control his hay fever), tolbutamide (to control his diabetes), a choleretic (to control his gallstones), and sulfamethizole. This last was news to Dr. Eisenstadt. He was aware that Warren's urologist had prescribed sulfamethizole at various times in the past. The sulfonamides have always (since their first appearance in the late nineteen-thirties) been the drug of choice in the control of infection in urinary-tract disorders. But now he learned that Warren had not confined his use of sulfamethizole to the periods immediately following his prostatic operations. He took the drug whenever he felt or feared a recurrence of prostatic pain. He sometimes took it every day. Dr. Eisenstadt opened his mouth to remonstrate, and then changed his mind. He didn't approve of this casual consumption of sulfamethizole, but he could see that it probably performed a salubrious psychological service. It was probably almost as necessary to Warren's well-being as any of his other drugs. Dr. Eisenstadt completed the examination in a generally optimistic frame of mind. For a man of Warren's age and afflictions, he was in satisfactory shape. The only problem was his hiccups. Their persistence was inexplicable. He may have been right in attributing Warren's first attack to a burst of indigestion. He may have been right in attributing the second to a little stroke. He may have been right in attributing others to the stresses and strains of surgery. And yet he didn't think so. He couldn't believe that so many different attacks had sprung from so many different sources. He couldn't believe in anything as arbitrary as that. He thought there was probably a single underlying cause. But he couldn't think what it might be.

Warren's hiccups lay unaccountably quiescent for just over a year. Then, in the spring of 1966, they unaccountably returned. The attack began on May 12. None of the usual home or office remedies had any prolonged effect, and on May 15 Warren was again admitted to St. Mary's Hospital for observation and treatment. The treatment included carbon-dioxide inhalation, intravenous injections of the respiratory stimulant pentylenetetrazol, and, finally, intravenous injections of a tranquilizer called chlorpromazine hydrochloride. The observation took the form of an allergy investigation. Dr. Eisenstadt was still convinced that all of Warren's hiccup attacks were the work of a common cause, and it now occurred to him that the cause might be some food, some drink, or some drug. The investigation followed the standard elimination procedure. Certain frequently allergenic foods — milk, eggs, corn, wheat — were successively eliminated from Warren's diet. Then, after an interval, they were successively and abundantly restored.

The results were noted. They were negative. Warren had no allergic reaction to any of the tested foods. Neither deprivation nor plenty had any effect on his hiccups. Dr. Eisenstadt then turned his attention to Warren's diet of drugs. The drugs that he took every day — digitalis, aluminum hydroxide, tolbutamide, antihistamine, the choleretic, and the diuretic — were one by one withdrawn. The results were the same as those of the food-allergy tests. Warren's hiccups continued. They continued through the elimination tests, they continued in spite of repeated carbon-dioxide inhalations, they continued in spite of the pentylenetetrazol injections. They were stopped at last by several commanding injections of chlorpromazine hydrochloride. That was on May 29, and Warren's endurance was almost at an end. He had endured three weeks of almost continuous hiccups.

The episode had also shaken Dr. Eisenstadt. It left him with an uneasy view of the future. Warren's persistent hiccups were becoming more and more persistent and less and less susceptible to treatment. He dreaded the next attack.

The next attack began on April 6, 1967. Warren was then making his home with a married daughter, and it was she who notified Dr. Eisenstadt. He responded by coming at once to the house. He found Warren exhausted and in bed — the hiccups had kept him awake all night — but otherwise much the same as before. His only notable bedside finding was that Warren was now wearing (on his urologist's prescription) an indwelling catheter to relieve his urinary difficulties. The hiccups were, as always, inexplicable. Dr. Eisenstadt considered his diminishing armamentarium, and gave Warren an intravenous injection of chlorpromazine hydrochloride. Chlorpromazine was the drug that he had used with success in the last persistent attack. Its effect this time was similarly, but not equally, successful. It lasted only overnight. Warren's hiccups then gradually returned — gradually and, as if some authoritative trace of chlorpromazine still lingered on, in a muted form. The spasms were weak and widely spaced. Dr. Eisenstadt prescribed an oral dose of Dramamine. The muted spasms subsided, but after a couple of restful hours Warren began to hiccup again. However, Dramamine was still effective, and it remained effective against a succession of recurring mild attacks. Then, on April 14, Warren was shaken by a violent seizure, and it was necessary for Dr. Eisenstadt to administer another chlorpromazine injection. That drug was once again effective, and Warren once again experienced an overnight remission and another week of generally mild and easily subdued attacks. By the end of the week, the Dramamine tablets had begun to lose their suppressive power, and Dr. Eisenstadt revised his prescription to Dramamine suppositories. This more forceful treatment prevailed for another week, and then it, too, began to weaken. On April 29, the violent hiccups violently reappeared. They yielded again for several hours to intravenous chlorpromazine, but when its hold relaxed they erupted as violently as before. Dramamine suppositories had no effect on this attack. It was brought under control with chlorpromazine in suppository form. But only momentarily. Another, more severe attack occurred on April 30, and this was followed three days later by another. That attack was intractable, and on Thursday, May 4, after two days of unbroken hiccups, Warren was admitted once more to St. Mary's Hospital. He reached there more dead than alive. Four weeks of almost continual jerking had exacerbated most of his chronic ailments, and his heart was enlarged and beating hard. He was groggy from lack of sleep, and weak from lack of food. The hiccups that kept him awake had kept him from eating, and he had lost some twenty pounds in weight. He was also in pain. All of his muscles were stretched and sore, and he hurt at every gulping, strangulated breath. His condition at admission was described as critical.

The first hospital attempt to hobble Warren's hiccups involved the once-triumphant carbon-dioxide-inhalation treatment. It gave him only a few short spells of relief. The next treatment was an intravenous injection of nikethamide. His hiccups continued unimpeded. A lumbar puncture was then proposed. A lumbar puncture is usually performed to obtain a quantity of cerebrospinal fluid for diagnostic analysis, but the operation was recommended now for therapeutic purposes as well. It was hoped that an examination of the fluid would suggest the cause of Warren's hiccups, and that the operation itself would excite a remedial reaction in the central nervous system. The lumbar puncture was half successful. It didn't explain the hiccups but it stopped them. The remission lasted twenty-four hours, and then the spasms started up again. Another lumbar puncture was tried, but this time nothing happened. Warren continued to hiccup. The news of his trouble had spread by now throughout the Jefferson County medical community, and on May 10 Dr. Eisenstadt was approached by a colleague who was also a hypnotist. The hypnotist offered Warren his salubrious powers of suggestion. Dr. Eisenstadt considered, and agreed. He didn't think that hypnotism would do much good. He didn't think that Warren's hiccups were psychogenically inspired. Psychogenic hiccups seldom interfere with sleep. But it could hardly do any harm. The hypnotist appeared at Warren's bedside at nine o'clock the following morning, and he stayed there most of the day. He then wrote a short memorandum and left it for Dr. Eisenstadt. It read, "Patient hypnotized and taught how to relax. Second technic: to forget how to hiccup. Third: improve bowel habits. Fourth: improve sleep pattern. The patient was very cooperative, and I feel that he responded well to hypnotherapy. He said he may want me to come back. Thanks for letting me see this fine gentleman." But Warren went on hiccuping. A desperate remedy composed of promethazine hydrochloride (an antihistamine), meperidine hydrochloride (or Demerol, a narcotic analgesic drug with certain antispasmodic powers), and oxygen inhalation produced a restful respite, but — as so often before — it was only temporary. Surgical intervention involving the phrenic nerves was next considered. That, however, wasn't possible here. The action of the diaphragm is directed by two phrenic nerves, and in Warren's unfortunate case both of these nerves were involved in his spasms. To block them both would also block his breathing. Dr. Eisenstadt and his hospital consultants consulted once again. There was almost nothing left to try. And then, while they were consulting, the crisis resolved itself. Warren's hiccups spontaneously stopped. His general condition at once began to improve, and on May 20, the seventeenth hospital day, he was judged sufficiently recovered to go home.

Warren was at home for just two days. He was discharged from the hospital on a Saturday, and on Monday he was readmitted. His hiccups had intractably returned. All of the standard remedies were tried, but only one was more than momentarily effective. That was oxygen, and even it gave only an hour or two of relief. Dr. Eisenstadt sat down with Warren's chart and reread its entries. The reading confirmed his belief that there were no more untried drugs to try. Nor were there any new techniques or devices. He reconsidered and once again discarded the possibility that Warren's hiccups might have their seat in one or another of his many chronic diseases. Except when exacerbated by the hiccups, all of Warren's diseases were pretty well under control. He reviewed the series of allergy tests that had been performed in 1966. The results still looked as conclusive as they had a year ago. There was nothing in Warren's diet that could possibly cause his hiccups. The same was true of the drugs he took. Dr. Eisenstadt checked them off — digitalis, aluminum hydroxide, tolbutamide, antihistamine, a diuretic, a choleretic, sulfamethizole. He stopped and looked again at the chart. Sulfamethizole was on the list of Warren's drugs, but it hadn't been included in the allergy tests. There had been no reason to suspect it. Its use was too occasional. It wasn't part of Warren's daily regimen. But now he began to wonder.

Dr. Eisenstadt returned the chart to the record room and went into the ward and had a word with Warren. Warren told him what he wanted to know. He was taking sulfamethizole. He had been taking it for the past two or three days. His prostate had been acting up again. Dr. Eisenstadt went to a telephone and put in a call to Warren's urologist. He explained what he had in mind. It wasn't a hunch. It wasn't even a notion. It was just that sulfamethizole was the only unknown factor, the only uninvestigated drug. The urologist listened, and unenthusiastically agreed to indulge Dr. Eisenstadt in his whim. He would see that Warren was taken off sulfamethizole for a couple of days. There were other, though less satisfactory, drugs that could replace it if the need arose. He would make the necessary arrangements at once. Dr.

Eisenstadt thanked him and crossed his fingers and waited. He wasn't kept in suspense for long. Warren was separated from sulfamethizole — from all and any sulfonamide drugs — in the late afternoon. Late the following afternoon, his hiccups began to subside. They continued to slow and slacken, and in the early evening of the second day they finally stopped altogether. The urologist extended the sulfonamide ban, and entered an antibiotic substitute in the order book. Another day went by, and then another. By the end of the week, it was certain. The attack was definitely over, and on Sunday, June 4, Warren was discharged to convalesce at home.

Warren's recovery left Dr. Eisenstadt in a state of hamstrung exultation. He thought he had found in sulfamethizole the root of Warren's endlessly recurring hiccups. The evidence was everywhere. Warren's last attack had followed a self-prescription of sulfamethizole, and the elimination of sulfamethizole had been followed by a remission. That plainly projected a cause-and-effect relationship between sulfamethizole and the hiccups. Nor was that all. The presence of sulfamethizole — or of some other sulfonamide drug — could at least be assumed in all of Warren's persistent attacks. Hindsight seemed to show that they had coincided with either self-prescription or surgical prescription of that drug. It was even possible to link it with Warren's first attack — the outbreak of hiccups that followed his hernia operation back in 1940. Nineteen-forty was before the development of antibiotics. The only drug then available for use in the routine prevention of post-operative infection was one of the sulfonamides. Reflection also suggested that sulfamethizole had the power as well as the opportunity to precipitate Warren's attacks. It was true that none of the sulfonamides had ever before been implicated in a case of persistent hiccups, but most of them were notorious for their manifold side effects, and these included a malevolent impact on the central nervous system. In a man as variously debilitated as Warren, that impact could easily detonate a violent attack of the hiccups. And yet none of this was proof. It was merely a structure of supposition. Warren's remission wasn't necessarily attributable to the elimination of sulfamethizole. It could have been simply spontaneous.

Whatever its nature, Warren's remission continued. He looked and felt and was in better health than he had been in for more than a year. His only remaining complaint was his perennially progressive prostatic hypertrophy, and toward the end of July the urologist judged — and Dr. Eisenstadt concurred — that his general condition was robust enough to withstand another transurethral re-resection. Warren reentered St. Mary's Hospital on July 24, and the operation was performed the next morning. The following day, Dr. Eisenstadt received a telephone call from the urologist. He was calling to report on Warren. The operation itself had gone very well, but now, he was sorry to say, a complication had developed. Warren had the hiccups again. He had been hiccuping for several hours and responded to none of the conventional remedies. Dr. Eisenstadt's heart sank. He thanked the urologist and said he would see what he could do and started to hang up — and had a sudden thought. The urologist was still on the line. By the way, Dr. Eisenstadt said. He spoke as casually as he could. What drug were they using to control post-operative bladder infection? Drug? the urologist said. They were using sulfamethizole. That was the usual drug in such . . . Memory struck him, and he stopped. He cleared his throat. But if Dr. Eisenstadt preferred, he would change his orders to some non-sulfonamide drug. As he had before. Dr. Eisenstadt said he thought it might be worth trying.

It was. Sulfamethizole was stopped and Warren's hiccups stopped, and he never took any more sulfonamides and he never hiccuped again.

# The West
# Branch Study

Dr. Stephen C. Schoenbaum arrived at West Branch (pop. 2,025), the seat of Ogemaw County, in northeastern Michigan, in a rented Ford sedan at about four o'clock on the afternoon of May 19, 1968. It was a Sunday afternoon, and raining. His first stop was at the Tri-Terrace Motel, on the outskirts of town. That part of Michigan is resort country, and the motel was built around a trout pond. He booked a room and left his luggage and asked the manager where he could get something to eat. He was directed to the Model Restaurant, near the traffic light on Houghton Avenue (or Route 76), the main street of town. He drove to the restaurant and had his supper, and then walked around the corner to the office of the District Health Department. Dr. Schoenbaum was an Epidemic Intelligence Service officer. He was twenty-six years old, he had just completed a year of intensive epidemiological training at the National Communicable Disease Center, in Atlanta, and this was his first field assignment. He had come up to West Branch (by plane that morning from Atlanta to Saginaw), in response to a request for help from the Michigan Department of Public Health in its investigation of an outbreak of infectious hepatitis that in just two weeks had grown from two to thirty-two cases.

Hepatitis is an inflammation of the liver. Its name defines its nature: "hepat" derives from the Greek for "liver," and "itis" is a Greek suffix meaning "inflammation." Many different agents, including drugs and chemicals, have the power to inflame the liver. Infectious hepatitis is one of two closely related inflammatory diseases of the liver that are confidently assumed to be of viral origin. The other is called serum hepatitis. These two varieties of hepatitis are by far the most common forms of the disease, and they constitute a public-health problem of ever-increasing concern throughout the Western world. In 1969, the most recent year of record, some fifty-five hundred cases of serum hepatitis and some forty-eight thousand cases of infectious hepatitis were reported in the United States. This would seem to present a total of around fifty-four thousand cases of viral hepatitis for that year, but public-health authorities read the record differently. It is their conviction that (for reasons of indifference or carelessness or misdiagnosis or subclinical infection) only a fraction of all cases of viral hepatitis that occur in this country are actually reported — probably only one in ten. They therefore read the record not as fifty thousand cases but as upward of five hundred thousand.

Until the middle nineteen-forties, when their differences were demonstrated by an international round of experiments involving human volunteers, infectious hepatitis and serum hepatitis were everywhere regarded as one and the same disease. It is not hard to understand why. They come on with equal abruptness, they produce identical signs and symptoms (chills, fever, lassitude, headache, loss of appetite, nausea, vomiting, abdominal pain, diarrhea, jaundice, prostration), and their impact on the liver is pathologically indistinguishable. They are also equally unresponsive to any specific treatment, and although full recovery (within two or three months) is the reassuring rule, both of them can permanently debilitate and sometimes even kill. They are not, however, identical. They spring from different viruses, and they are differently disseminated. Infectious hepatitis is usually transmitted by direct person-to-person contact or by food or water contaminated with the excreta of an earlier victim. Serum hepatitis is less conventionally, and less easily, spread. The virus of serum hepatitis lodges not in the gastrointestinal system but in the blood stream, and it can be conveyed only by an inoculation of infected blood. In addition to (and perhaps because of) these different modes of transmission, the different viruses establish themselves and multiply at different rates of speed. Infectious hepatitis generally manifests its presence about thirty days after exposure. In serum hepatitis, the incubation period ranges from three weeks to three or four months. An attack of hepatitis, like an attack of any viral disease (poliomyelitis, smallpox, measles, whooping cough) produces in its surviving victims an immunity to future infection. But the immunities conferred by infectious hepatitis and serum hepatitis are separate and distinct. An attack of infectious hepatitis protects against a second attack of infectious hepatitis but not against an attack of serum hepatitis, and serum hepatitis also protects only against itself. It is this fact — the fruit of a hundred painful human experiments — that makes it certain that infectious hepatitis and serum hepatitis are, at bottom, different diseases.

The avoidance of the viral hepatitides, despite their immunological potential, is very largely a matter of chance. Medical science has not yet succeeded (as it has with smallpox and poliomyelitis and measles and so many other viral diseases) in developing a protective vaccine. It is far from certain that it ever will. There is a formidable reason for this. The development of a vaccine begins with the laboratory cultivation of the relevant pathogen, and to the best of current knowledge the viruses of human hepatitis are parasites so specialized that they can grow and proliferate only in a living human cell. A reliable passive protection against infectious hepatitis is offered by gamma globulin. Gamma, or immune, globulin is a blood protein extracted from the pooled blood of at least ten thousand donors that (because many of these donors will have had infectious hepatitis) contains infectious hepatitis antibodies. The force of an attack of infectious hepatitis can be bridled and held to a subclinical, or unapparent, infection by an injection of gamma globulin given soon after probable exposure. The effectiveness of gamma globulin, however, is limited to this prophylactic role, for antibodies thus acquired are quickly (in four or five weeks) metabolized and dismembered. The effectiveness of gamma globulin is limited also to infectious hepatitis. Serum hepatitis does not seem to lend itself to gamma-globulin prophylaxis. Why this should be is uncertain. One suggested reason is that serum hepatitis is insufficiently common for its antibodies to be powerfully present in the ten-thousand-donor pools.

Infectious hepatitis has a natural history as long as that of any of the many epidemic diseases. There is no reason to doubt that its origins go back at least five thousand years, to the first coming together of men in city, or community, life. It is thought to have been glimpsed as an entity as early as the Hippocratic era, and it has certainly long been known (under such names as "field jaundice" and "camp jaundice") as a major military scourge. It has been recorded (by army surgeons) as a serious source of misery in every war since the Napoleonic Wars. Serum hepatitis has no such lineage, and its history is anything but natural. It is one of a growing number of upstart diseases that have been brought into being by a triumphant medical technology. Although it probably first appeared when man first learned to puncture his skin for religious or cosmetic purposes, serum hepatitis came into prominent medical view only with the development of smallpox vaccination, and it has mounted to its present eminence with the extension of that procedure to other diseases, and with the invention of the blood transfusion and the hypodermic syringe. Serum hepatitis very seldom occurs in epidemic form. Its rigid epidemiology inhibits its rapid spread. The few large outbreaks of serum hepatitis on record have chiefly stemmed from either blood-bank blood contaminated by infected donors or from slipshod immunization programs, and most of these have involved military or institutional personnel. Serum hepatitis most commonly occurs in occasional cases of insidious origin (its generally long incubation period makes retrospective explication difficult), and its typical appearances are almost always the result of a disregard of elementary hygiene.

162

In 1961, a New Jersey osteopath infected some forty patients by not bothering to autoclave or otherwise sterilize the syringe he used for drug injections. More recently, in 1969, a girl was infected in a Larchmont jewelry store when she had her ears pierced with an unwashed communal punch. And the promiscuous tattoo needle has over the years produced almost as many cases of serum hepatitis as it has epidermal declarations of patriotism and filial love. But these are not typical victims. The typical victim of serum hepatitis in the United States these days is a phenomenon as grimly specialized as the disease itself. He is a young heroin (or amphetamine) user who shares a syringe with a friend. Serum hepatitis would thus seem to be, as Dr. Michael B. Gregg, chief of the Viral Diseases Section of the National Communicable Disease Center, has put it, "a public-health problem compounded by a sociological problem."

The typical victim of infectious hepatitis is a more prosaic person. He can be anyone confronted by a victim or who eats a contaminated meal or takes a drink of contaminated water. Not much (in the absence of a scrupulous universal cleanliness) can be done to protect him. The only defensive procedure possible is to block the spread (or a recurrence) of a discovered outbreak by finding and stopping its source and immunizing potential victims. That, however, is well worth doing, and that was Dr. Schoenbaum's job in West Branch.

Dr. Schoenbaum was received at the West Branch office of the District Health Department by the District Health Officer. She was Dr. Ophelia Baker. Her husband, Dr. Thomas Baker, one of five physicians then practicing in West Branch, was with her. The Bakers led Dr. Schoenbaum into Dr. Ophe-

163

lia's office and gave him a cup of coffee and brought him up to date on the epidemic.

"It was still going," Dr. Schoenbaum says. "Seven new case reports had come in since Saturday. They raised the total from thirty-two to thirty-nine. There had been no deaths, and none was expected, but there were a couple of patients sick enough to be hospitalized. They were in the local hospital — the Tolfree Memorial Hospital. A gamma-globulin program had been started five days ago, on May 14, and the contacts of all the known cases were being inoculated. The epidemic was definitely an epidemic. Dr. Ophelia got out her records. Only seven cases of hepatitis had been reported in the preceding twelve months in the whole of Ogemaw County. There was as yet no epidemic curve — no chronological pattern. The data needed to draw it — the dates when the victims first became sick — were lacking. Dr. Ophelia had been too busy with the gamma-globulin program. It was quite a program. It ran almost two weeks, and they ended up immunizing something over seven thousand people. The information on the reported cases was the standard minimum — name, address, age. The cases were of both sexes, they seemed to live all over the county, and they ranged in age from five to thirty-nine. There was one moderately interesting fact. A majority of the cases were teen-agers, and most of them were boys. I didn't know what that signified, and I didn't try to guess. I simply copied off the names and addresses. All of them would have to be seen and interviewed. The results of the interviews would set the course of the investigation. I hoped they would, anyway. I knew there weren't any shortcuts. I could only hope that the truth would emerge from the evidence.

"I met with Dr. Ophelia again on Monday morning. The rain

was over, and it was a fine spring day. We met by prearrangement at the hospital, and she introduced me at rounds to
the other West Branch physicians. They gave me a very
warm welcome. They were overworked and tired, and apparently under some pressure from the community. The point
appeared to be that Ogemaw County is a summer-resort area,
and a continuing epidemic could be bad for business. Also, I
guess, a lot of the working population was laid up sick. We
left the hospital, and I suggested to Dr. Ophelia that maybe I
ought to have a look at the schools. There were two of them,
and she took me around and I met the principals. One of the
schools was the public school — a consolidated, all-grades
school with an enrollment of around fifteen hundred. The
other was a small Roman Catholic school. Both schools were
within a block or two of the Houghton Avenue business district, and both were served by the same school buses. We then
went on to Dr. Ophelia's office. It was almost ten o'clock and
time for her to get back to the gamma-globulin program. The
District sanitarian was waiting for us at the office. He's a very
nice fellow named James Hasty. Mr. Hasty knows everybody
in West Branch and almost everybody in Ogemaw County,
and Dr. Ophelia had arranged for him to guide me around on
my interviews and generally smooth my way.

"We took right off in my car. The family I wanted to call
on first was a West Branch family I'll call Simpson. It was the
largest family on the list, and it had the largest number of
cases. I thought that might make for an instructive start.
There were eight in the family — the parents, four boys (including twelve-year-old twins), and two girls. The children
ranged in age from five to fifteen. Five of the children and
Mrs. Simpson were sick. Only Mr. Simpson and one of the

165

twins had escaped the epidemic. The Simpsons lived on the edge of town. Mrs. Simpson was in bed, too sick to see me, but Mr. Simpson happened to be at home. He and the five sick children told me what they could. There was municipal water in West Branch, but the Simpsons pumped their water from a private well. They bought milk from one or another of the Houghton Avenue stores, usually the A & P. They did their marketing at the same stores. They occasionally bought something at the West Branch Bakery, and they occasionally had a meal or a snack at one of the restaurants or one of the Dairy Queen drive-ins. There were two Dairy Queens in Ogemaw County — one in West Branch and one about twelve miles out of town on the Rose City road. None of the family had recently attended any large gathering at which food or drinks were served. Hepatitis was the only recent illness in the family. The children all were pupils at the public school. I took a sample of water for laboratory analysis, and then got down to the individual cases. What I wanted now were the onset dates of illness — when the first symptoms appeared. This was the essence of the interview. The onset date minus thirty days would give me the approximate date of exposure. We take thirty days as the average incubation period in infectious hepatitis. Mr. Simpson went upstairs and talked to his wife and came back with a calendar, and he and the children worked out the dates. The onset dates for the two girls were May 3 and May 4. The boys — all three of them — took sick on May 5. Mrs. Simpson's first symptoms appeared four days later, on May 9. Well, that was a start. Those six dates made a kind of pattern. If the Simpsons were in any way typical, the epidemic had its beginning in early April.

"They seemed to be entirely typical. Mr. Hasty and I made

three more calls that day, and I interviewed four more patients. One was a boy of eleven whose history almost exactly paralleled that of the three Simpson boys. His illness, like theirs, had begun on May 5. He too attended the public school. He occasionally had a meal with his parents at one or another of the Houghton Avenue restaurants, he sometimes had a snack at one of the Dairy Queens, and his parents traded at the A & P and most of the other food stores, including the West Branch Bakery. His history differed from that of the Simpsons in only one respect. The family water was municipal water. Two of the three other patients were a woman of thirty-nine and her eight-year-old daughter. She had become sick on May 11 and her daughter on May 10. The daughter attended the Catholic school. Their histories otherwise were substantially the same as the rest. The last patient I interviewed that afternoon was a man — a bachelor of thirty. He was a salesman. His illness had begun on May 13. That suggested that his exposure had occurred on April 13, but his records suggested an earlier date. They showed that he had been out of town between April 11 and April 13, and from April 15 to April 20. April 14, the one day in that period when he had been in West Branch, was a Sunday, and he had spent it at home. His general history, with one exception, was much like that of the others. It included municipal water, the A & P and other markets, the restaurants, and the two Dairy Queens. The exception was the West Branch Bakery. He said he never set foot in the bakery. He and the owner had quarreled. I thought about that on the way back to the office. I had practically decided that water and milk could be eliminated as likely vehicles of infection here. And now I thought maybe we could drop the bakery too. I mentioned this to Mr. Hasty.

He agreed about water and milk. The community was about equally divided between municipal water and private wells, and all the milk came from sources outside the county. But about the bakery — the fact that the salesman never traded there didn't really mean very much. The bakery was more than just a store. It also supplied bread and pastries to most of the markets in town, and to all of the restaurants.

"I talked to Atlanta that night. I didn't have much to report, but they had some news for me. They were sending me some help. He was a fellow EIS officer named James M. Gardner. Gardner was between assignments. He had just finished an assignment at the Michigan State Public Health Department, down in Lansing, and he wasn't due to report for his next assignment — in California — until the following Monday, so they had asked him to spend the interval up here with me. He arrived on Tuesday morning. I hadn't asked for help, but I was glad enough to have it. I got gladder as the week went on. Eight more cases were reported on Tuesday, four more came in on Wednesday, and on Thursday there were six. That brought the total number of cases in West Branch and the rest of Ogemaw County up to fifty-seven. It would have taken me two weeks to see that many people, but with Gardner to help it only took three days. By Thursday night, we had seen and interviewed all the West Branch cases and most of those in the outlying county. The results were all we had hoped for. They were even more than that. We got a good epidemic curve. It was virtually the same as our final curve. It showed that the epidemic began with a single case on April 28, built to a peak of thirteen cases on May 12, and then dropped to a final case on May 20. All but five of the cases had had their onset between May 2 and May 14. This clustering was very instructive. It indicated the time of exposure — around the middle of the first half of April. It established what we had only assumed before — that all of the cases were infected by the same source. They were too close together to be related in any other way. And it told us that the epidemic was either ending or already over. But that wasn't all. Those were merely the formal results. We learned some even more interesting things in our travels around the county. One of these was that the epidemic might be wider in scope than any of us had supposed. Several people we talked to had friends or relatives living elsewhere who had been in West Branch recently and who now were sick with hepatitis. Or so they said. We also heard and confirmed that there had been some hepatitis in the community about a month before the epidemic began. There were two cases in particular. One was a girl who worked at the Rose City Dairy Queen. She left work sick on April 4. The other was a man I'll call John Rush. Rush was a baker at the West Branch Bakery, and he took sick on April 6.

"We sat down with Dr. Ophelia on Thursday night and had a conference. The question was what to do next. There was an embarrassment of promising possibilities. Talk to Rush? Talk to the girl? Look into those outside cases? And we still had a few more county cases to see. We decided to let the county cases wait. They couldn't tell us much that we didn't already know. Rush and the girl were a different matter. They were very interesting news. Either one of them could be the index case — the source case of the epidemic. They both were sick at the right time, and they both had jobs that had to do with food. The girl's job was especially provocative. She made us think of a recent classic case — an epidemic in Morris County, New Jersey, in 1965 that was traced to contaminated strawberry sauce in an ice-cream drive-in. But, of course, that wasn't enough. Our histories showed that everybody seemed to patronize the Dairy Queens, but they also showed that everybody seemed to patronize the bakery, too. We needed something stronger than suspicion. We needed something that would narrow the field a bit. That brought us around to the outside cases. A visitor to West Branch would probably have fewer contacts than a resident. There was one presumably outside case within reasonable reach. She was a schoolteacher I'll call Miss Brown, and she lived in the village of Au Gres, on Saginaw Bay, about thirty miles southeast of West Branch. We decided she was worth an immediate visit. Our information was that she had been in West Branch recently. It could be very helpful to find out when and where.

"The three of us drove down to Au Gres the next morning. That was Friday, May 24. Dr. Ophelia was able to come along because the gamma-globulin program was just about over. She was determined to be in on Miss Brown. She had the same feeling that Gardner and I had that this could give us a lead. You may wonder why we didn't just pick up the telephone and give Miss Brown a call. The reason is this. The epidemiological experience has been that telephone interviews are seldom satisfactory. A telephone conversation is too abrupt, too remote. People make more of an effort when they're talking face-to-face. So we paid Miss Brown a visit. She was sick, but not too sick to see us. There was no doubt about its being hepatitis. She was still icteric — still jaundiced. Dr. Ophelia handled the introductions. Her presence was invaluable. She helped Miss Brown to relax and think back and remember. Miss Brown's memory was excellent. As a matter of fact, it was exhilarating. The chronology of her illness placed her squarely in the epidemic. Her onset date was May 5. It was true that she had been in West Branch recently. She had stopped there twice in the past three months — on March 20 and again on April 5. But only very briefly. On the first occasion she had a cup of coffee in one of the restaurants. That was all — just a cup of coffee. She was sure of the date because her mother had died the day before and she was on her way across the state to Petoskey for the funeral. Petoskey was her home town. She drove back to Au Gres on March 23, but this time she didn't stop at West Branch. She was also sure about her second West Branch visit. April 5 was a Friday and the beginning of spring vacation, and she was driving to Petoskey again to spend the holiday with her father. It was late afternoon, and she was hungry. She stopped in West Branch and went into the bakery there and got something to eat on the way. She bought some pastry — a piece of coffee cake and three cupcakes with yellow Easter-bunny icing. That definitely was on her way to Petoskey. It couldn't have been on her return. She returned on April 14, and April 14 was a Sunday — Easter Sunday. We thanked Miss Brown and marched out to the car and headed back to West Branch. We sang all the way."

Miss Brown's emphatic testimony marked the end of the floundering phase of the West Branch study. It also marked the end of Dr. Gardner's participation in the investigation. He left on Saturday for his new assignment in California. Dr. Schoenbaum was alone again, but again for only a day. He spent that day on a final round of interviews. Four more cases had been reported since Thursday. That brought the epidemic total up to sixty-one. By Sunday night, however, he had histories on them all. His new reinforcement arrived on Monday. He was an EIS officer on loan from the Shelby County Public Health Department, in Memphis, named E. Eugene Page, Jr. Dr. Schoenbaum and Dr. Page spent Monday afternoon and evening at the Tri-Terrace Motel reviewing the collected case histories. They spent Monday night at the West Branch Bakery.

"We got there around midnight," Dr. Schoenbaum says. "That was when their baking day began. They baked six nights a week — Sunday through Friday. I had already talked to the owner and made the necessary arrangements, and he was there to meet us and show us around. I had explained the nature of hepatitis and told him what we knew about the epidemic. I told him that it unquestionably stemmed from a common source, and that we had some evidence that the source might be his baked goods. One of his people, as he knew, had been sick with hepatitis back in April, and he could be what we called the source case. Our evidence wasn't proof, but it was enough to require an investigation of the bakery. We wanted to see how the baking was done. We wanted to see if bakery goods could be a source of infection. The owner was extremely cooperative. He could very easily have been hostile and difficult. In return, I assured him that we wouldn't publicize our visit. We would keep it a secret until the end of the investigation. There was no chance that anybody would see us arrive. West Branch is asleep by midnight.

"He let us in the back door. The back room was the baking room. There were two bakers — the head baker and Rush. The owner was also a baker by trade, but he didn't do much baking anymore. Only when they were shorthanded. He worked days in the shop up front, and after introducing us, he left and went home. Page and I stood around and watched the bakers work. They were mixing dough. There was a bread dough and a pastry dough. They mixed them separately, but they mixed them both by hand. They did everything by hand — mixing, kneading, shaping. Even when they used a mechanical mixer, they scooped the dough out by hand. Rush was older than the head baker, and he was nice and friendly, but he didn't look very bright. But he seemed to know his job. We watched them, and it was interesting for a while, and then it began to get boring. It also began to seem like a waste of time. Rush and the bakery was our one big hope. The Dairy Queen girl had just about dropped out of sight. The case histories made her very unlikely. When we checked them over carefully, it turned out that her Dairy Queen wasn't as popular as we had thought. It was the other Dairy Queen that most of the people went to. She might have been the source of a case or two, but she couldn't be the epidemic index case. That was Rush. Or so we thought until we watched the baking. He had every opportunity to contaminate the dough, but the dough was only the beginning. It then went into the oven and baked for half an hour or more at a temperature of at least three hundred and fifty degrees. Thirty minutes at anything much over a hundred and thirty degrees will kill the virus of infectious hepatitis.

"But we stayed and watched. They made some doughnuts — fried cakes, they called them — and cooked them in boiling oil. Our hopes got dimmer and dimmer. They offered us some of the fried cakes, and Page ate a couple. I declined. I don't know why exactly. There wasn't any risk. Rush was fully recovered, and the head baker had never even been sick. I said I wasn't hungry. I really wasn't — I couldn't have eaten anything anywhere just then. The time dragged on. Around three-thirty, they finished baking and emptied the ovens and stacked the bread and rolls for sale in the shop up front or for delivery to the store and restaurant customers. The next step was icing and glazing the pastry. Some of the frostings were already cooked and ready to use, and some they made without cooking. They started in by glazing the fried cakes. The glaze was in a five-inch pan about five feet long. What they did was take a double handful of cakes and dip them in the glaze and turn them over and around and then lift them out and line them up on a rack. That was glazing. That was the entire process. But it was a revelation to us. Page and I were wide awake in a minute. The process was much the same with the other kinds of pastry. I remember at one point Rush was up to his elbows in glaze. He piled a load of fried cakes on the rack, and then turned and walked across to another counter and started icing cupcakes. He didn't bother with a pastry tube. He used his hands — the same bare hands he had used on the fried cakes. He scooped up a handful of icing and squeezed it out through his fingers. He was an expert. He did a beautiful job. It was horrifying. Page and I could hardly keep from shouting. They called the West Branch Bakery a home bakery. What they should have called it was a hand bakery.

"Rush was almost certainly the index case. We watched and asked questions, and by five o'clock, when we finally called it a night, we had everything we needed but proof. Rush had had every opportunity to contaminate the pastry, and also had had the capacity. His understanding of hygiene was very primitive. Baking was the only protective process. Anything that was contaminated after that would stay contaminated forever. Watching Rush work, we began to wonder when the contamination might have occurred. Did it happen on a succession of nights? Or on a single night? We found that a single contamination could even account for people being exposed over a period of several days. The head baker told us that unused glazes and icings were carried over from one night to the next. He said they often used leftover glaze to start a new batch. We also learned that the bakery regularly sold day-old pastry as well as day-old bread. And not only that. Unsold pastry was often frozen and sold a few days later. The hepatitis virus can be killed by freezing, but not that kind of freezing. A few days isn't long enough. It takes a year or more. All of those points were persuasive. We began to incline toward the idea that the contaminated pastry was contaminated in the course of a single night. It actually seemed more probable than a series of accidents — even for a man like Rush. The night that seemed most probable was the early morning of Friday, April 5. It was supported by the clustering of onset dates, and by Rush's own experience. April 6 was the day he consulted a doctor — the apparent date of onset. But he had obviously been infectious at work that Thursday night and Friday morning.

"There was only one way to pin it down. We would have to interview the cases again. If we were right about Rush and the bakery, the proof would be forthcoming. We would find that all of the victims had consumed some iced or glazed pastry from the West Branch Bakery between Friday, April 5 and the end of the following week. The period could be a bit open-ended, but it had to begin on April 5. That was the day — the only day — that Miss Brown had visited the bakery. Page and I didn't do much work on Tuesday. We slept until early afternoon. At some point, I had a call from Atlanta. They were sending up a distinguished foreign visitor to observe our methods. His name was Zdenek Jezek, and he was a senior WHO medical officer stationed at Ulan Bator, in Outer Mongolia. He arrived that evening. I remember his greeting. 'I am Jezek of Czechoslovakia,' he said. So he was a Czech. That was a little disappointing. We had been expecting a Mongolian. As a matter of fact, he was a thorough Czech. We briefed him on the epidemic, and when we came to the age and sex distribution of the cases, he shook his head. There was something wrong. Teen-age boys didn't eat pastry. Not in Czechoslovakia. Bakery customers were women and young children. He couldn't believe that things were different in Michigan. He thought it over, and then announced that he would get the facts by conducting an investigation of his own. All we had to do was arrange for him to sit somewhere out of sight in the bakery and record exactly who came in. I thought that might be interesting, and I said I would make the arrangements, but maybe he ought to wait a day or two and get his bearings first. I suggested that he sit in with Page and me on our new round of interviews.

"We began on Wednesday morning, and we began with the out-of-county cases. They would be the quickest way to determine if we were moving in the right direction or completely wrong. This time we worked by telephone. We had to. There were thirteen substantiated cases, including Miss Brown, and all of them were out of easy reach. Two were even out of state — a man in Indianapolis and another in Wethersfield, Connecticut. The first case we called was a man in Mount Pleasant, about fifty miles to the south. He confirmed that he had hepatitis. The onset date was May 3. Yes, he had been in West Branch, and in early April — April 5 through April 7. He and his wife had driven up to attend a wedding. We knew about the wedding, and none of the principals or other guests was on our epidemic list. He and his wife had eaten all of their meals with the other wedding guests. He stopped and thought a minute. Except on the day they arrived. That was April 5, and he dropped in the West Branch Bakery and bought four iced cupcakes. Which he ate. He wasn't a teen-ager — he was twenty-two — but he ate them all. I don't know what Jezek made of that. But I do know that Page and I began to feel very good.

"The other out-of-county cases told the same fascinating story. It was fantastic. There were two married sisters from Detroit with four children who spent three days in April — April 8 through April 10 — in a cottage in the woods about ten miles out of town. On the morning of April 9, one of the women drove into West Branch alone to mail some letters, and brought back half a dozen fried cakes from the West Branch Bakery for lunch. Three of the cakes were glazed and three were plain. The two women and one of the children ate the glazed cakes, and they were all three sick with hepatitis. Two became sick on May 7 and the other on May 11. The three other children were well. I talked to the man in Connecticut. I ran him down in a hospital. Yes, he had hepatitis. Yes, he had been in West Branch. It was his home town and he had been there to visit his mother. He arrived on April 4 and left on April 6. On April 5 or April 6, he wasn't sure which, he had dropped into the West Branch Bakery to see the owner. They were old friends. The owner gave him a couple of glazed doughnuts, and he ate them while they talked. The man in Indianapolis was like the group from Detroit. He spent three days — April 7 through April

9 — at a cottage down at Clear Lake, and on Monday, April 8, he came into town to get his shoes repaired. While he was waiting, he walked into the West Branch Bakery and bought a piece of iced Danish pastry. A thirteen-year-old boy from Roscommon County was in town on April 5 — and so on. Every one of the out-of-county cases confirmed the place, the date, and the vehicle.

"We still had the community cases to question. There was no real doubt in our minds about the answers we would get, but we had to make the effort. We had to be thorough and sure. Most of what is known about viral hepatitis has come from epidemiological studies, and every careful study can be a contribution. There was also Jezek and his bakery survey. I introduced him to the bakery owner, and they worked out the details — the logistics. Jezek is a small man and they found a little corner where he could sit unnoticed behind a showcase and have a view between the shelves of all the comings and goings. He spent a full day there — from seven in the morning until the bakery closed at six o'clock that night. His findings were useful. They combined with the information that Page and I were getting to explain the big teen-ager clientele. He found that adults — mostly women — were in and out of the store all day. Very few young children — children under ten — ever came into the bakery, and then only in the late afternoon. The teen-agers showed up in a body at noon and again after three o'clock. The reason, as our interviews showed, was very simple. The teen-agers were, of course, high-school kids, and the high-school kids were allowed to leave the school grounds for lunch. The younger kids — the grade-school children and all of the children at the parochial school — had lunch at school.

Jezek's tabulations showed that the bakery was a favorite teen-ager place for lunch. Almost half of the customers he counted in his survey — ninety-six out of a total of two hundred and fourteen — were teen-agers. Moreover — and this again confirmed our information — they all bought pastry: glazed fried cakes, iced cupcakes, chocolate éclairs, frosted twists, iced brownies. That and a Coke or something seemed to be the popular lunch. The only difference between Jezek's findings and our epidemic data was that his teen-agers were about evenly divided between girls and boys. I have no idea what that means — if it means anything. Maybe the girls were dieting back in April. But it seemed to satisfy Jezek.

"The second series of community interviews took about a week. We finished the job on Monday, June 3. We tidied up and said our good-byes on Tuesday, and on Wednesday we left for home. The total number of cases in the epidemic turned out to be seventy-six — sixty-three in West Branch and Ogemaw County, and thirteen in Detroit, Indianapolis, Wethersfield, and elsewhere. We managed to interview all but one of the local cases. The only one we missed was a man who was away on a trip of some kind. We ended up on Monday night, and the place we ended at was exactly where I had started on that Monday morning just two weeks before — with the Simpson family. With Mrs. Simpson, actually. She was now fully recovered and able to see us. It was very strange. I mean, if I had known the right questions to ask, I might almost have solved the whole problem on that first visit. This is what Mrs. Simpson told me. On Saturday morning, April 6, she went marketing, and on the way home, she stopped at the bakery and bought some pastry — an assortment of glazed fried cakes and iced cupcakes. She was sure of the date because she remembered hurrying home to watch the news on television. Martin Luther King had been assassinated on Thursday, and there had been riots in Memphis on Friday and she wanted to see if the trouble was still going on. Mr. Simpson was working, but the two daughters were at home. Mrs. Simpson and the girls sat down at the television and they each ate a cupcake while they watched the program. After a while, the two oldest boys came in, and they helped themselves to some pastry. Then the twins arrived. There was only one piece of pastry left — a fried cake. They saw it and made a grab, and the one I'll call Jerry lost out. He didn't get any pastry. And he was also the twin who didn't get hepatitis."

# A Woman
## with a Headache

A woman I'll call Mildred Anderson — Mrs. Harold
Anderson — was admitted to Temple University Hospital, in
North Philadelphia, on the afternoon of Friday, January 19,
1968, for observation and treatment of a severe and persistent
headache. Mrs. Anderson's admission was arranged by Dr. Albert J. Finestone, an internist and a clinical professor of medicine at Temple University School of Medicine, to whom she
had been referred by her family physician, and she was shown
to a two-bed room on the fourth floor and made as comfortable
as possible. That was around two o'clock. At five, an intern on
Dr. Finestone's service named Mary E. Moore dropped in for
the opening diagnostic interrogation.

Dr. Moore introduced herself. She sat down and smiled and
asked Mrs. Anderson how she felt. Mrs. Anderson said she

felt pretty good. She hesitated. As a matter of fact, she felt fine. It was a funny thing, she said. It was almost embarrassing. Her headache was gone. In the two or three hours that she had been in the hospital, it had completely vanished. She didn't understand it at all. It was almost as if the hospital had scared it away. Dr. Moore said nothing. She nodded and made a sympathetic sound. But she thought she understood it well enough. Dr. Moore is not only a doctor of medicine. She is also a doctor of philosophy in experimental psychology, and she knew that it was entirely possible that Mrs. Anderson's headache *had* been scared away. Hospitals often have that effect on functional, or psychogenic, disorders. That didn't mean, however, that Mrs. Anderson's headache *was* functional in origin. It was just a possibility. Hospitals often momentarily exert much the same inhibiting effect on the pain of disorders that are fully and ferociously somatic.

Dr. Moore got out her pen and a ruled personal-history form. Mrs. Anderson was a striking-looking woman. Her hair was white, her complexion was rough and florid, and her eyes were large and expressive. She was small and notably thin. Her age, as given on her chart, was forty-one. The chart also noted that she and her husband, a civil engineer, were childless, and owned their own home. Mrs. Anderson shifted her position in bed — and Dr. Moore was startled to see that her spine was twisted and bent in the humpbacked conformation known as kyphoscoliosis. Startled and interested. That explained Mrs. Anderson's size, and possibly more than that. Dr. Moore began the interview. Mrs. Anderson was quietly and politely responsive. Her chief complaint was, of course, a headache. It had first appeared about three weeks ago. She had suffered off and on for many years from what she believed were migraine headaches, but this was nothing like those. There was no nausea, no vomiting, no sensitivity to light. It was simply an excruciating pain that progressed from the back of her head to the top. The migraine headaches had begun in childhood, and she was the only member of her family to be so afflicted. The only drug she ever took was aspirin — until recently. Three weeks ago, her doctor prescribed a drug called Fiorinal for her headache. Dr. Moore nodded. Fiorinal is a popular, nonnarcotic sedative and analgesic. However, Mrs. Anderson said, it hadn't done much good. This was the first real relief she had had in all those weeks. It was also her first experience as a hospital patient. Her back was not the result of either illness or injury: she had been born that way. She had never been seriously ill, and she had no known allergies. She drank occasionally, but she didn't smoke. Her ruddy complexion was normal for her. Her skin was naturally very dry. It was often blotchy, and it tended to redden whenever she was tense or nervous. She had been like that all her life. Was she nervous now? Well, yes — she supposed she was. After all, she had never been hospitalized before.

That completed the historical phase of the interview. Dr. Moore moved from her chair to the bedside, and began the customary routine physical examination. She identified Mrs. Anderson's chronic dermatitis as ichthyosis congenita. She found Mrs. Anderson's eyes, ears, nose, throat, and neck to be essentially normal. There was no ocular evidence of brain tumor or of any intracranial swelling, and no venous distension, and no thyroid- or lymph-gland enlargement. She confirmed her snap diagnosis of kyphoscoliosis. Mrs. Anderson's breasts were normal. Her heart was normal in size and rhythm, and her lungs were clear to auscultation and percussion. There were no discernible abdominal masses, and her liver and spleen felt normal. Her reflexes were satisfactory, as were the results of a careful neurological examination. Dr. Moore added these reassuring but unilluminating findings to the record. She then turned to the order sheet and noted down the several preliminary tests and studies that she wished to have made. They included blood analyses (hematocrit, hemoglobin, serology, blood sugar, kidney function), urinalysis, chest X-ray, spine X-ray, neck X-ray, skull X-ray, brain scan, electroencephalogram, and electrocardiogram. The results of one or another of these should produce at least a glimmer of diagnostic enlightenment. Dr. Moore also asked that a dermatologist be consulted about the treatment of Mrs. Anderson's ichthyosis. She further noted that Mrs. Anderson was to be given codeine as needed (thirty milligrams every four hours) for the relief of her headache, and Nembutal (one hundred milligrams) for sleep. She closed the preliminary report with a preliminary comment: "Impression: (1) Congenital kyphoscoliosis. (2) Congenital ichthyosis. (3) Headache of unknown etiology — probably cervical spine deformity as cause. To be ruled out: Brain tumor or other intracerebral lesion."

Mrs. Anderson spent a generally comfortable night. She slept with the help of Nembutal, but she had no need for codeine. Her headache was still ambiguously quiescent. She was rested but not yet fully relaxed when Dr. Finestone walked in on his rounds the following morning with his entourage of students and interns. Dr. Finestone was roughly familiar with the nature of her case. He had spoken with Dr. Moore the night before, and he had just now read her notes and comments. Nevertheless, like all scrupulous attending physicians, he sat down and saw for himself. He led Mrs. Anderson briefly back through her relevant history, and then appraised by direct examination what her history suggested were the physical essentials. He was interested and puzzled by the disappearance of her headache. But he could see no cause for any alarm, and he ended the visit with a word of sincere reassurance.

The next day — January 21 — was a Sunday. It passed agreeably for Mrs. Anderson. She had a visit from her husband, and there was still no return of her headache. An intern on weekend duty noted that she seemed less tense and restless than reported the day before. The strangeness of hospital life appeared to be wearing off. On Monday, the first results of the diagnostic studies were reported. They included the standard laboratory tests, the electrocardiogram, and three of the four requested X-ray examinations — chest, neck, and spine. Dr. Finestone and Dr. Moore went over the findings together. None of the reports contained any diagnostic surprises. Mrs. Anderson's chest, heart, kidneys, and blood were normal. The radiologist's report on the look of her neck and spine read: "A marked degree of scoliosis of the dorsal spine with the convexity to the right is seen. . . . Changes in the thorax secondary to scoliosis are also noted. The cervical and dorsal spine reveal no other significant abnormalities. The intervertebral foramina are patent. No osteolytic or osteoblastic abnormalities are seen." (Osteolysis is a dissolution of bone, and an osteoblast is a cell involved in bone production.) Later that day, the dermatological consultant confirmed that Mrs. Anderson's skin condition was indeed a congenital ichthyosis, and prescribed for its correction a regimen of oil baths and rubs.

Two of the three remaining studies were completed on Wednesday. They were the skull X-ray and the electroencephalogram. Dr. Finestone recorded the results on Mrs. Anderson's chart: "EEG & skull films negative." He then added his comments and conclusions: "Pain gone. Likely diagnosis — cervical spondylosis. Doubt intracranial cause." The results of the brain-scan study were reported the following day. They considerably decreased the possibility of any cerebral involvement: "Following administration of technetium 99m pertechnetate, the brain was examined by the scintillation camera in five views (anterior, posterior, left lateral, right lateral, and vertex) after preparation with potassium perchlorate. No abnormalities are noted in any of these views." That was the last of the diagnostic studies, and it seemed to Dr. Moore almost conclusive. It strengthened her impression that there was nothing very wrong with Mrs. Anderson. Even the woman's headache was gone — spontaneously gone — and had been gone for close to a week. Dr. Moore noted on the chart for Dr. Finestone's approval that Mrs. Anderson was now ready for discharge. Dr. Finestone concurred in this judgment, and Mrs. Anderson was discharged from the hospital early on Thursday afternoon. Her case was closed with a final diagnosis: "Headache secondary to cervical scoliosis and nervous tension."

Dr. Moore was with Mrs. Anderson when her husband arrived to take her home. Mr. Anderson was much like his wife — quiet, pleasant, cooperative. He was also, like his wife, a little confused and worried. They didn't understand that equivocal week in the hospital. Dr. Moore undertook to reassure them. She reminded Mrs. Anderson of the many tests and examinations that she had undergone. They were the reason for her protracted hospital stay. She then explained their uniform results. There was no cause for any concern. Just the reverse. The tests had made it clear that Mrs. Anderson was in enviably excellent health. Dr. Moore tried to speak with conviction, and the Andersons were convinced. They thanked her and shook her hand and left the hospital arm in arm. Dr. Moore went on to her other patients. Some of them might never be discharged, and Mrs. Anderson dropped untroubled from her mind.

Dr. Finestone was the first to have Mrs. Anderson recalled to his attention. She was returned to his mind at one o'clock on Friday afternoon by another telephone call. The call reached him at Temple University Hospital, and the caller was Mr. Anderson. He was apologetically distraught. He was calling about his wife. When he had brought her home from the hospital on Thursday afternoon she seemed to be in good spirits and she said she was feeling fine. He left her at home and went down to his office to finish up some urgent work. When he got back to the house a couple of hours later, she was prostrate on the sofa with one of her terrible headaches. He telephoned their doctor, and the doctor came to the house and gave her an injection of Demerol. That helped her through the night. But the headache came back this morning, and now — just a few minutes ago — his wife had fainted. He had come home from his office for lunch to see how she was. She told him she was feeling sick and dizzy, and that was when she fainted. She was conscious now, but she looked as if she might pass out again any minute. What should he do? Dr. Finestone asked if he had called the family doctor again. No? Then Mr. Anderson should call him, and right away. He was their regular doctor, he lived in the neighborhood, and he had treated Mrs. Anderson only the night before. However, if Mr. Anderson couldn't reach the doctor, he was to call Dr. Finestone again and bring his wife to the hospital. Mr. Anderson thanked him, and Dr. Finestone hung up and resumed his interrupted rounds. He wondered what could have happened to Mrs. Anderson. He couldn't relate it to anything in her known condition of health. It was very strange. It almost sounded hysterical. But she hadn't impressed him as being that neurotic. He finished his rounds, and Mr. Anderson still hadn't called. It was safe to assume that the matter was now in the hands of the family doctor. He looked around for Dr. Moore. It would be interesting to hear her opinion. But she wasn't on the floor. Dr. Finestone went down and changed out of his long white coat and put on his overcoat and went home. He didn't see Dr. Moore again until Sunday. By then it was all over.

Dr. Moore was assigned to overnight duty on Saturday. She reported to the hospital at noon and spent the afternoon on the floor. There were old patients to see and new patients to meet and study. She had dinner in the hospital cafeteria at five o'clock, and then went back to continue with her patients and see them settled for the night. It was an undemanding evening on her floor, and around midnight she went down to the emergency room and joined a couple of other idling interns and the resident on duty there. She had been sitting in their company about an hour — smoking and talking and drinking coffee — when she heard herself being paged. She walked around the corner to the house telephone. The call was not a summons from her floor. It was an outside call. The caller was a young woman and her voice was shrill and excited.

"Is this Dr. Mary Moore?"

"Yes."

"I'm the niece of Mrs. Anderson. One of her nieces. I think you helped take care of her when she was in the hospital?"

"That's right."

"Well, I'm over here at her house. At the Andersons' house. I came over this evening because my uncle called and asked me to help, and something terrible has happened to her. It's awful. She had this terrible headache yesterday, and she passed out I don't know how many times — and now she's lost the power of the tendons in her legs."

Dr. Moore stood silent with the telephone in her hand. She was stunned. She couldn't believe it. Mrs. Anderson had spent a full week under careful observation in a first-class university teaching hospital, and according to the most sophisticated tests and tabulations she was in essentially the best of health. There had been no sign of any serious ailment. But now — just two days later — she ...

Dr. Moore took a deep breath. "You mean she's paralyzed?"

"I guess that's what it is," the niece said. "She's lost the power of her tendons."

"I think I'd better speak to Mrs. Anderson. Can you get her to the phone?"

"I'm afraid you can't. I mean, it wouldn't do any good. She isn't making any sense."

"Then let me speak to Mr. Anderson."

"My uncle?" She gave a wild laugh. "He's acting just as crazy as she is."

"Oh," Dr. Moore said. But she also felt a kind of relief. If both of the Andersons were affected, it must be something that had happened after Mrs. Anderson left the hospital. It might be some deranging form of food poisoning. It might be drugs. It might be simple alcohol. She remembered that Mrs.

Anderson liked an occasional drink. "Do you think they might be drunk?"

"I don't know," the niece said. "I don't think so. I don't see any glasses or bottles or anything." She gave another wild laugh. "My uncle fainted this afternoon. That was before he called me."

Dr. Moore hesitated. She wondered if the niece had been drinking. "How about you?" she said. "Are you all right?"

"I don't know," the niece said. "I guess so. Sure, I'm OK."

"I hope so," Dr. Moore said. "I want your aunt and uncle at the hospital as soon as possible. Can you get them here? Do you need any help?"

"I don't need any help. My friends have a car. I've got some friends here with me. I guess I forgot to tell you that. They're an older couple I know."

"All right," Dr. Moore said. "Come to the emergency room. I'll meet you there."

"OK," the niece said.

Dr. Moore waited at the emergency-room door. It opened and closed on the regular Saturday-night procession of beatings and knifings and car-wreck lacerations. At a little past two, the car with the niece and her friends and her aunt and uncle pulled into the curb, and Dr. Moore sent an orderly out to meet them with a rolling stretcher. She watched him lifting Mrs. Anderson onto the stretcher and the rest of them milling around and trying to help. Mr. Anderson wore striped pajamas under his overcoat, and he seemed to be yelling. The orderly pushed the stretcher up the walk and into the foyer, and Mrs. Anderson lifted her head. Her face was red and her eyes were bright. She saw Dr. Moore, and let out a cry of delight.

"Hi, there, Dr. Moore," she said. "I never expected to see you again. How you doing?"

"I'm fine," Dr. Moore said. "But what about you? What happened?"

Mrs. Anderson laughed.

Dr. Moore asked the niece and her friends to wait, and nodded to the orderly. She led the stretcher down the hall and into an examination booth. Mr. Anderson came stumbling loudly after them. His face was as flushed as his wife's. He flopped down on a chair and leaned loosely back. Dr. Moore sat down on a stool and looked at them. She felt she didn't know them at all. They didn't act or talk, or even look, like the Andersons she knew. She could only think they were drunk — or drugged. But she couldn't think what drugs they might have got to make them act this way. And they didn't smell of liquor.

"All right," she said. "Now tell me what happened. Have you been drinking?"

"Drinking?" Mrs. Anderson said. "Certainly not."

"We haven't been anything," Mr. Anderson said, and laughed.

"You haven't eaten anything unusual?"

"I haven't eaten hardly anything."

"Or taken any drugs?"

Mrs. Anderson let out a wail.

"Then tell me what happened."

"It was my head," Mrs. Anderson said. "You know about my headaches. Well, I got this terrible —"

"Now, wait a minute," Mr. Anderson said. "Wait just a minute. That isn't quite the way —"

"What isn't the way? I think I know —"

"But you're getting it all wrong. It wasn't —"

"Be quiet."

"Don't you tell me to be —"

"I said be quiet."

"Shut up."

"Stop it," Dr. Moore said. "Both of you. There's no reason to get so excited." She considered. They were obviously in no immediate danger. She decided to let the questioning go for a moment. They might be calmer then. And she wanted a moment to organize her own ideas. She stood up. "I'm going to leave you for a minute. Try to relax. I'll be right back."

Dr. Moore went down the hall to the house officers' corner. The resident was with a patient, but there were still two interns there. She told them about the Andersons.

"I just don't know what's going on," she said. "There's something wrong with these people. They're out of their heads. But I don't know why. The only other thing is her face is awfully red. Except that her face is always red." She stopped. "You know, I just realized something. Her husband's face is also awfully red. They've both got bright-red faces."

One of the interns cocked his head. "Like cherry red?" he said. "Like carbon-monoxide poisoning?"

"My God," Dr. Moore said. "My God — that's it."

The cause of carbon-monoxide poisoning is the inhalation of carbon-monoxide gas. Carbon-monoxide gas is generated by the incomplete combustion of some carbonaceous (wood, coal, petroleum) material. Complete combustion, however, is not a natural phenomenon. It occurs only under the most fastidiously controlled conditions. Thus, for all practical purposes, carbon monoxide is a regular product of fire. Its nature is as insidious as its generation. The presence of carbon monoxide in a room or a street or an automobile is impossible to detect by any means naturally available to man. Its anonymity is as total as that of air. Carbon monoxide is colorless, odorless, and tasteless. It even has the same specific gravity as air. It neither sinks to the ground nor rises away like smoke but mixes and mingles indistinguishably with the atmosphere.

Carbon monoxide, though always dangerous and often deadly, is a poison only in the language of convenience. It is actually an asphyxiant. It deprives its victims of the oxygen they breathe by displacing oxygen in the carrier hemoglobin of the red blood cells. This suffocating displacement is easily accomplished. Hemoglobin, by some hematological quirk, much prefers carbon monoxide to oxygen. Recent investigators have mathematically rendered its preference into odds of approximately three hundred to one. Their calculations suggest that a given concentration of carbon monoxide in the air can successfully compete for the molecular embrace of hemoglobin with anything up to three hundred times its concentration of oxygen. The result of the eager union of carbon monoxide and hemoglobin is a brilliant-red compound called carboxyhemoglobin. Carboxyhemoglobin is the source of the characteristic cherry-red flush of carbon-monoxide poisoning. It also, however, has more sinister powers. It inhibits the release of whatever oxygen has managed to combine with hemoglobin. Carboxyhemoglobin is a stable compound, but its bonds are far from unbreakable. They readily loosen under the impact of abundant oxygen, and the hemoglobin so released, unharmed by its impetuous encounter, is free to resume its proper physiological functions. That providential frailty of carboxyhemoglobin simplifies the treatment of carbon-monoxide poisoning. It is often treatment enough to remove the victim from the poisoned air. A few hours of rest will then restore the normal chemistry of his blood. More seriously stricken victims can usually be rallied by the administration of pure oxygen under pressure. Unless, of course, they are already dead or dying.

It takes very little carbon monoxide to contaminate the air. The virulence of carbon monoxide is very nearly unique. A concentration of only two one-hundredths of one percent (or two hundred parts of carbon monoxide per million parts of air) can kindle in a couple of hours a dull frontal headache, and an exposure of just five minutes to air containing one percent of carbon monoxide is almost invariably fatal. Moreover, the action of carbon monoxide is ferociously quickened by such environmental factors as heat and altitude, by the presence of debilitating diseases like anemia and asthma, and by physical activity. The blood of a man at labor becomes saturated with carbon monoxide about three times faster than that of a man at rest. Mild but perceptible symptoms of illness ordinarily appear when the carboxyhemoglobin level approaches twenty percent. More conspicuous symptoms — severe occipital headache, nausea, vomiting, dizziness, muscular incoordination, disorientation — develop as the saturation mounts toward forty percent. At fifty percent, unconsciousness usually descends, and a saturation of sixty-six percent (or the conversion of two-thirds of the body's supply of hemoglobin into carboxyhemoglobin) is classically considered fatal.

The sources of carbon monoxide are abundant in the urban Western world. In the United States, they are almost everywhere. Carbon monoxide is perniciously present in the effluvia of all internal-combustion engines, most industrial plants, and many mines, mills, and workshops. There are also many domestic sources: unvented space heaters, floor furnaces, kerosene stoves, gas ranges, camp stoves, and blocked or faulty flues. Among the more familiar fuels, manufactured gas is potentially doubly dangerous, for it not only produces carbon monoxide (like natural gas and the other carbonaceous materials) but actually contains it. Burning charcoal is especially rich in carbon monoxide — so rich that in France, where charcoal fires are widely used for cooking, carbon-monoxide poisoning is sometimes called *folie des cuisiniers*. Another rich source is burning tobacco. The blood of heavy cigarette smokers (those who smoke two or three packages a day) has been found to contain as much as ten percent carboxyhemoglobin, or almost enough to cause manifest signs of illness. The most insidious source of carbon monoxide is, of course, the gasoline engine. It is also, with an ever-increasing multitude of ever more powerful automobiles on the streets, an increasingly serious one. Automobile (and motorboat) exhaust fumes contain about seven percent carbon monoxide, and where traffic is slow and heavy the amount of carbon monoxide pumped into the air can easily approach a toxic level. A field study undertaken by the National Air Pollution Control Administration in 1967 has demonstrated that it often does. The study was conducted in ten cities (Atlanta, Baltimore, Chicago, Cincinnati, Detroit, Louisville, New York, Minneapolis, Denver, and Los Angeles) at the peak of the rush-hour traffic. Bumper-to-bumper speeds produce about three times as much carbon monoxide as a cruising speed of forty-five miles an hour. Instruments mounted in a test car analyzed the air at the level of the driver's head. The findings ranged from a low (in Louisville)

195

of sixty-six parts of carbon monoxide per million parts of air to a high (in Los Angeles) of one hundred fifty-one parts of carbon monoxide per million parts of air. Concentrations of one hundred or more were recorded in four of the other cities: Cincinnati (100), Detroit (120), Minneapolis (134), and Denver (142). New York and Chicago both showed concentrations of ninety-five. The maximum allowable concentration of carbon monoxide for an exposure of several hours (established by the American Standards Association around 1900) is one hundred parts per million parts of air. Within the past few years, however, many investigators have come to believe — on the basis of certain studies on human volunteers which demonstrate that even minute concentrations of carbon monoxide can subtly dull the crucial sense of time and distance — that a concentration of one hundred is much too high for perfect safety, and they have proposed that the maximum be lowered to fifty. In the Soviet Union, the legal (though not necessarily enforced) maximum is eighteen.

It was once generally held that carbon-monoxide poisoning occurred in both acute and chronic forms. Most investigators now deny the possibility of a chronic form of carbon-monoxide intoxication. They distinguish instead between acute and chronic exposure. "Chronic exposure does not produce chronic poisoning," Dr. David H. Goldstein, professor of environmental medicine at New York University Medical Center, noted in a 1963 medical textbook, "but, rather, repeated episodes of mild acute poisoning. Intermittent day-to-day exposures are not cumulative in effect." The incidence of severe acute carbon-monoxide poisoning has declined in the United States in recent years. This is largely attributable to the widespread installation of safety devices (fans, baffles, alarm meters) in industrial plants, and to safer home appliances. In New York City, for example, a total of four hundred twenty cases of serious carbon-monoxide poisoning (a hundred thirty-one of them fatal) was reported in 1951. The total for 1967 was seventy-three cases, of which four were fatal. Most of these cases were the consequence of dilapidated equipment, sitting in a closed car with the engine running, or a deliberate, suicidal exposure. Less conspicuously clinical cases, on the other hand, are almost certainly increasing. There are no real records of such cases, because they are seldom recognized and reported, but it is probable that thousands of Americans suffer some degree of carbon-monoxide poisoning — a late-afternoon headache, a little lurch of nausea, a creeping irritability — every day. The victims are unsuspecting people who regularly expose themselves to air that, through ignorance or indifference or inadvertence, is perennially polluted. They include automobile mechanics, parking-garage attendants, traffic policemen, newspaper-kiosk keepers, cabdrivers, urban-bus drivers, janitors, commuting motorists, and, every now and then, a housewife like Mildred Anderson.

Dr. Moore couldn't doubt that the Andersons' trouble was carbon-monoxide poisoning. She went back to the examination booth in a euphoria of relief. Carbon monoxide answered every question. It explained Mrs. Anderson's interminable headache, it explained the disappearance of the headache after a few hours in the unpolluted air of the hospital, it explained the return of the headache, and the dizziness, the faintness, the weakness, the bizarre behavior. It had to be carbon monoxide, and the source could only be something in the Anderson house. Something that was regularly but intermittently in use.

Something like a kitchen range, a hot-water heater, a furnace. That would also explain why Mr. Anderson had only now become sick. He hadn't been sufficiently exposed; he had only been home at night until this weekend began.

"I couldn't doubt it was carbon monoxide," Dr. Moore says, "but I couldn't, of course, just assume it. I had to be sure. I had to document it. There was a senior medical student I knew hanging around, and I grabbed him and asked him to draw some blood from the Andersons for a carboxyhemoglobin-determination test. Meanwhile, I got them both breathing pure oxygen. Then I thought of the niece. I remembered how funny she had sounded. So I rounded her up and got her on oxygen, too. Then I called the lab. The technician who could do the test I wanted wasn't on duty. I got permission to call him at home, and I called him and he moaned and groaned and carried on, but he finally got dressed and came over. A carboxyhemoglobin-determination test takes about twenty minutes, and in twenty minutes we had the confirmation: Mr. Anderson's carboxyhemoglobin level was thirty-nine percent, and Mrs. Anderson's was thirty-seven.

"By the time we got the lab reports, the Andersons were both pretty well recovered. But I kept them at the hospital. I couldn't send them back to that contaminated house. The niece threw off her little touch of poisoning very fast, and I talked to her and her friends before they left. I arranged for them to take the Andersons in until their house had been inspected. They told me the Andersons used natural gas for heating and cooking, and that the house had seemed awfully hot and a little smelly of what they now decided was gas. They said they would get in touch with the gas company the first thing in the morning. I heard the rest of the story a couple of days later.

Mrs. Anderson called me. An inspector from the gas company had come out and made a thorough investigation, and my hunch had been in the right direction. The trouble was the furnace. Or, rather, the furnace flue. The inspector had found it practically blocked with fallen bricks. Mrs. Anderson thought she knew how that had happened. They had had their chimney repaired several months before — sometime back in the summer. It had needed pointing. And apparently the mason who repaired it also managed to drop a few old bricks down the flue."

# A Small,
# Apprehensive Child

Her experience was so exceptional that I'll give her an unexceptional name. I'll call her Barbara Logan. Barbara was then — in the late spring and early summer of 1968 — six and a half years old. She lived with her mother, a recent divorcée, in a two-family house in the City Park section of Denver, and it was there, at around eight o'clock on the night of June 9, a Sunday, that her experience began. It began with fever and a spasm of vomiting. She vomited off and on all night. She vomited all day Monday. She vomited all through Monday night. On Tuesday morning, she was still hot to the touch (Mrs. Logan didn't have a clinical thermometer), and she complained for the first time of pain. Her throat was sore, she said, and there was a sore place under her left arm. Mrs. Logan felt and found a lump about the size of a golf ball. It was hard and painfully tender. That alarmed her. She got Barbara up and into some clothes and telephoned for a taxicab. Mrs. Logan had no regular physician. She told the driver to drive them to Children's Hospital. That was the hospital nearest her home.

The driver, after a glance at Barbara, delivered them to the hospital emergency room. The physician on duty there, a woman, briefly questioned Mrs. Logan, and then turned her attention to Barbara. Her findings, which she noted on the standard chart, confirmed the cabdriver's snap impression: "Physical examination revealed an acutely ill child. Eyes sunken. Looks very miserable. Surprisingly cooperative. Lips and nailbeds cyanotic. Two-inch roughly round left axillary node which is very tender. Mild generalized abdominal tenderness. Joints not hot or swollen. Right eardrum red. Throat slightly infected. Chest clear. Slight tachycardia [pulse rate], 120. No [heart] murmur. Neck supple. Appears dehydrated. Temperature, 104.4." This last — almost six degrees of fever in so crowded a clinical context — was decisive. The physician made the necessary arrangements for Barbara's immediate admission. She also arranged for certain indicated laboratory tests (blood analysis, urinalysis, throat culture) and a chest X-ray. She did not attempt a comprehensive diagnosis. She merely noted the several apparent infections: otitis media (inflammation of the middle ear), gastritis, and pharyngitis. And added: "Rule out pneumonia."

Barbara was led up to a ward and put to bed. She was wrapped in a cool sheet to temper her fever and given a mild analgesic for comfort. An antibiotic regimen to curb her apparent infections was begun: two hundred thousand units of penicillin every four hours, and four hundred milligrams of sulfisoxazole every eight hours. Half an hour later, she vomited. Then she seemed to feel better, and presently fell asleep. The following day, her condition was, at best, equivocal. The results of the chest X-ray were within normal limits, and any threat of pneumonia appeared to be remote. Her white-blood-cell count, a standard index of infection, was only slightly elevated (to 8,300 per cubic millimeter), and the differential (or constituent) count was essentially normal. The intern assigned to the case noted on her chart: "Temperature, 100. Hydration improved. Patient extremely fussy. Nodes in axilla have increased 3-fold in nite to 15 x 10 cm. mass, which is exquisitely tender. She has had no more vomiting. Taking oral fluids. Primary culture of urine, blood & throat shows no growth. I am not impressed by her response to antibiotic therapy at this time. Will do second blood culture & watch closely."

A week went by. Barbara's condition remained uncomfortably equivocal. On Monday, June 17, the intern noted: "Still very tender in axilla, but swelling is down. First blood culture grew Gram-negative rods at 4 days. Second blood culture negative at 5 days. Still has temperature 100." His second entry was a clouded clarification. A rod is a bacillus of cylindrical (or rod-shaped) conformation, and a Gram-negative rod is one that reacts negatively to a staining test developed by the early-twentieth-century Danish investigator Hans Christian Joachim Gram. This reaction is a primary characteristic of numerous bacteria. Some, though only some, of these are pathogenic to man. That group, however, includes the agents of brucellosis, glanders, gonorrhea, influenza, plague, salmonellosis, shigellosis, tularemia, typhoid fever, and whooping cough. Later that day, the intern noted on the record that the cryptic Gram-negative presence in Barbara's blood had been delivered to the nearby laboratory of the Colorado State Health Department for dispatch to the Laboratory Branch of the National Communicable Disease Center, at Atlanta, for definitive screening and precise identification. He then returned to the bedside with a sudden, discordant note: "Patient spiked temperature to 103.4." Confronted by this inscrutable turn, he reinforced the standing regimen with two new varieties of penicillin — potassium phenoxy-methyl and sodium methicillin. The following day he requested an X-ray examination of the left shoulder "to rule out possibility of osteomyelitis." The thought had apparently struck him that a fitful inflammation of the bone might be responsible for both Barbara's persistent fever and the equally stubborn swelling under her arm. If so, his mind was quickly put at rest. The roentgenologist reported on Wednesday morning that he could find no evidence of any bone involvement. Barbara's condition that morning was also reassuring. "Patient feels better," the intern noted. "Ate good breakfast. Tenderness in L. axilla diminished considerably." The sudden improvement continued. Barbara's fever fell to a scant 100 degrees. She continued to eat with appetite, and the tender swelling under her arm continued to subside. On Friday, for the first time, her temperature dropped to normal. She continued free of fever for the next four days, and on Tuesday morning, June 25, the intern closed his record of the case. "Temperature still normal," he noted. "CBC [complete blood count] WNL [within normal limits]. Patient to be discharged today." She was discharged that afternoon, with a comprehensive supply of sulfisoxazole and supporting penicillins, to convalesce at home.

Barbara's convalescence was a fleeting one. It barely lasted over Tuesday night. She awoke on Wednesday morning with a familiar pain in her armpit. The swelling there had reappeared, and the area was now so sensitive that it hurt to even close her arm. Mrs. Logan was more confused than alarmed. Barbara, after all, had just been discharged from the hospital as recovered from whatever had ailed her. She felt Barbara's forehead. It was reassuringly cool. And Barbara said she was hungry. That surely meant there was nothing seriously wrong. She decided to wait and see. She waited until Thursday afternoon. Barbara was still cool and still able to eat with appetite, but she was also still in pain. Mrs. Logan called a cab and took her back to the hospital. "Glands in axilla have increased," the emergency-room physician noted. "Now is developing enlarged nodes in left side of neck. Child does not look well. Appetite good & no fever since discharge. To return next Wednesday." Barbara did not, however, return the following Wednesday. Mrs. Logan returned her the following day. The enigmatic swellings had increased again in size and sensitivity. "Looks very poorly," the examining physician noted, and revising his Thursday opinion, he arranged for her readmission. "Suggest surgical consultation for possible incision & drainage." Her temperature then — at eleven o'clock in the morning — was 101.4.

Barbara was assigned this time to a bed in a ward for infectious diseases. She was visited there around noon by an intern on that service. He found her to be "a small, apprehensive child with a painful, swollen left axilla" and confined his diagnosis to the merely descriptive: "Left axillary lymphadenitis." Her indifferent response to antibiotic therapy impressed him even less than it had the intern earlier in attendance. He expressed his dissatisfaction by canceling the earlier orders. That was the usual step. The next was to mount a new and more aggressive antibiotic attack. But there he stopped, uncertain. The discarded assault was standard in what appeared to be the circumstances of the case. He reflected, and then (with the approval of the guiding resident) stepped in a different direction. Barbara, until further orders, was to be given no medication at all. The nature of those orders would depend upon the nature of the organism that had been cultured from her blood. He would wait until the report on that came through from Atlanta. It was not an easy decision, and it was not an easy wait. Barbara's condition continued as before. Her temperature returned mysteriously to normal and the painful swellings persisted. June ended and July began. On July 2, the operation proposed by the admitting physician was successfully performed, and it had, as planned, the immediate salubrious effect of reducing the monstrous glands. The following day, at two o'clock in the afternoon, the report at last came through: The intern noted it on the record: "CDC called to report blood culture of 6/11/68 as suspect of *Pasteurella pestis.*" That most emphatically answered his question. He could now proceed to treatment with the confidence of certainty. But it far from closed the case. *Pasteurella pestis* is the causative agent of plague.

Plague, as its prototypical name so starkly proclaims, is the oldest and most dangerous of the great epidemic diseases. The weapon with which the Lord punished the Philistines for their victory over the Israelites (and for their acquisition of the Ark of the Covenant) is generally identified as plague. Most medical historians believe that plague was probably the chief constituent of the ambiguous "Plague of Athens" described by

Thucydides in his *History of the Peloponnesian War*. It was plague that ravaged the Byzantine Empire in the time of Justinian (around A.D. 542) and, according to the contemporary historian Procopius, killed half of the population. And it was plague that practically decimated Europe in the Black Death pandemic of 1348. Its appearances since then have been less dramatically lethal, but the disease is still far from conquered. Plague was more or less endemic in Europe from the fourteenth century to the end of the eighteenth century (an epidemic in Prussia in 1709 took well over three hundred thousand lives), and it still prevails in its classic epidemic form in much of Asia (including Vietnam), and in parts of Africa and South America. It is one of only four diseases that are still accepted by public-health authorities throughout the world as quarantinable. The other diseases whose presence aboard a ship or a plane is sufficient cause to quarantine the craft are cholera, smallpox, and yellow fever.

No disease has inspired a larger general literature than plague. Its literary fruits alone include the *Decameron* of Boccaccio, Daniel Defoe's *A Journal of the Plague Year*, and *The Plague*, by Albert Camus. The contagion from which the characters in the *Decameron* have fled to a hilltop palace near Florence is the Black Death, and Boccaccio's generally accurate description of the disease at its most relentless indicates the origin of that lurid medieval name. "In men and women alike," he notes, "there appeared at the beginning of the malady, certain swellings, either on the groin or under the armpits, whereof some waxed to the bigness of a common apple, others like unto an egg, some more and some less, and these the vulgar named plague-boils. From these two parts the aforesaid death-bearing plague-boils proceeded, in brief space, to appear and come indifferently in every part of the body; wherefrom, after awhile, the fashion of the contagion began to change into black or blue blotches, which showed themselves in many first on the arms and about the thighs and after spread to every other part of the person, and in some large and sparse and in others small and thick-sown; and like as the plague-boils had been first and yet were a very certain token of coming death, even so were these for everyone to whom they came."

The black or blue blotches of the Black Death are multiple tiny hemorrhages of the skin, and occur in both of the two chief forms of plague. These forms are known as bubonic plague and pneumonic plague. Bubonic plague is the classic and the commoner form. It takes its name from the inflammatory swellings (so obvious to Boccaccio and so mysterious to the doctors attending Barbara Logan) of the lymphatic glands in the groin and the armpit. These traditionally definitive swellings are called buboes, from the Greek *boubon*, for groin. Pneumonic plague, as its name declares, is plague in which the lungs are involved. Essentially, it is a complication of untreated bubonic plague. Until shortly after the Second World War, when an effective antibiotic treatment for plague was found in streptomycin and tetracyclines, pneumonic plague was a common consequence of bubonic plague. Untreated bubonic plague is fatal in about fifty percent of cases. Untreated pneumonic plague is always fatal. When plague is promptly and properly treated, however, prompt recovery is the reliable rule. Bubonic plague, though easily capable of the greatest epidemic spread, often occurs sporadically. Pneumonic plague is wholly an epidemic disease, and its appearances are invariably preceded by an outbreak of bubonic plague.

Few diseases have been more portentously explained than plague. Its cause was once (perhaps originally) believed to be a baleful conjunction of the planets Saturn, Jupiter, and Mars. It was also thought (perhaps alternatively) to be caused by other cosmic events — comets, volcanic eruptions, earthquakes. Another, and less fortuitous, explanation attributed plague to the machinations of Jews ("It was believed that the Jews had poisoned the wells," Guy de Chauliac, physician to Pope Clement VI, noted in his contemporary account of the pandemic of 1348, "and they killed them."). A more persistent view envisioned plague as one of the sterner manifestations of the Wrath of God. This attractively guilt-ridden concept (which inspired the wild-eyed peregrinations of the Flagellants in the fourteenth century) was widely embraced until almost the modern era. Even physicians accepted it, though usually with reservations. A pious seventeenth-century German physician named Johannes Raicus attempted to clarify the matter with a scholarly tract. There were, he pronounced in 1620 in his *Ex Flagello Dei*, two different sources of plague. One was divine in origin and the other was a natural visitation. Divine plague, being a punishment inflicted for cause on a discovered sinner, was not infectious. The other was.

By "infectious," Raicus meant "contagious." The truly infectious, or bacterial, nature of plague was demonstrated independently by the Japanese bacteriologist Shibasaburo Kitasato and by Alexandre Yersin, a French investigator, during an epidemic of the disease in Hong Kong in 1894. Another French investigator, Paul Louis Simond, is celebrated as the discoverer of its contagious, or communicable, nature. Simond suggested, in a report to *Annals de l'Institut Pasteur* in 1898, that the *Pasteurella pestis* of Kitasato and Yersin is not among man's natural microbial enemies. It was his correct assumption that plague is primarily a disease of rats that is accidentally conveyed to man by a variety of fleas. Moreover, as he proposed and as subsequent investigators were able to establish, these fleas prefer the blood of rats to that of man, and it is probable that they turn to man only when rats are scarce. Outbreaks of plague in man tend to follow directly upon a decimating epidemic of plague among rats. (The seventeenth-century French painter Nicolas Poussin precociously included among the panicking crowds in his graphic portrayal of "The Plague of the Philistines" the bodies of several dead rats.) The manner in which the flea transmits *P. pestis* to man is also accidental. A flea that has fed on an infected rat ingests a multiplicity of plague bacilli. These bacilli accumulate and eventually block the forestomach of the flea, and in order to swallow newly gathered blood, it is forced to regurgitate. Much of this bacilli-laden vomitus inevitably passes into the bloodstream of the host. Plague produced by the bite of a contaminated flea is bubonic plague. Bubonic plague cannot be transmitted by ordinary contact from one human victim to another. Pneumonic plague can. Its accompanying coughs and sneezes are as irresistibly infectious as those of the common cold.

Simond's report on the role of the rat in human plague, like most such pathfinding studies, was at first dismissed as absurd. It then was acclaimed as definitive. It is now merely recalled as a milestone. For there is more to plague than Simond could suppose in 1898. More recent investigation has shown that plague is not, as he conceived, exclusively a rat-borne disease of seaport cities — the morbid consequence of the arrival in a rat-infested city of a rat-infested ship. That is only its classic approach, and one that an almost universal insistence on rat-proof ship construction is rapidly rendering historic. The susceptibility of the domestic rat to plague is now known to be shared by many other wholly undomesticated rodents and rodentlike animals. Some seventy equally prolific and comparably flea-ridden creatures — including mice, rabbits, hares, voles, ground squirrels, prairie dogs, marmots, chipmunks — are more or less hospitable to *P. pestis*. There are pockets of wild-rodent, or sylvatic, plague in the wilds of China and Southeast Asia, in Africa, and in North and South America. One of the biggest of these enzootic reservoirs lies in the American West. In fact, it *is* the West. The area in which infected animals (and their attendant fleas) have been found embraces the states of Washington, Oregon, California, Nevada, Utah, Idaho, Montana, North Dakota, Wyoming, Arizona, New Mexico, Colorado, Kansas, Oklahoma, and Texas.

Plague is generally thought to have entered the United States with a pack of ailing rats that climbed ashore from a burning freighter on the San Francisco waterfront. Opponents of this notion suggest that plague was present here long before its presence was formally noted. San Francisco, at any rate, was the scene of the first American epidemic. The epidemic began with the discovery of a dead Chinese in the rat-infested basement of the Globe Hotel in Chinatown on March 6, 1900, and it lasted, largely because the local authorities tried to hush the matter up, for almost four years — until February of 1904. It was one of the deadliest epidemics on record. One hundred and twenty-one people were stricken, and all but three of them died — a mortality rate of ninety-seven percent. A second, and only somewhat less lethal, epidemic occurred in San Francisco in 1907, the year after the earthquake and fire. Three other American cities have experienced serious outbreaks of plague — Seattle, also in 1907; New Orleans in 1914 and again in 1919; and Los Angeles in 1924. The Los Angeles epidemic was the last recorded appearance in this country of classic, urban, rat-borne plague. It was not, however, the last appearance here of plague. Since 1908, when an epizootic in ground squirrels near Oakland, California, abruptly announced its presence, sylvatic plague has seized, along with numberless rodents, a number of human victims. One hundred and twenty-three cases, sixty-seven of them fatal, are known. Eighty-three (or two-thirds) of these have occurred in the past thirty years, and more than half of those recent victims have been children. Twenty-five of them — like Barbara Logan — were less than nine years old.

The telephoned report on the nature of Barbara Logan's illness that Denver Children's Hospital received on the afternoon of July 3, 1968, was one of three identically alerting calls that were made that day by the Laboratory Branch of the National Communicable Disease Center, in Atlanta. The others went to Dr. Cecil S. Mollohan, chief of the Epidemiology Section of the Colorado State Department of Health, in Denver, and to a station of the Ecological Investigations Program of the United States Public Health Service at Fort Collins, Colorado. This last call was taken by Dr. Jack D. Poland, then acting chief (he is now the head) of the station's Zoonoses Section. A zoonosis is a disease of animals that may be conveyed to man. There are many such diseases, and the

Zoonoses Section is professionally familiar with almost all of them, but the zoonosis with which Dr. Poland and his staff are principally concerned is plague. He expressed this concern in a matter of minutes with a telephone call to Denver.

Dr. Poland says: "I called Dr. Mollohan. That isn't the way it's usually done, of course. I should have waited for him to call me. The protocol in public health is that a federal agency comes into a local matter on invitation from the local authority — the city or county or state — in charge of the investigation. But we don't stand much on ceremony with plague. I knew Dr. Mollohan would see it that way, and he did. He needed and wanted our help. I told him I'd get our people on it right away. Fort Collins is sixty miles from Denver, but that's no distance in this part of the world. Then I remembered. I said I'd do better than that. I said it so happened that Harry Hill was in Denver that day on a routine tick-fever job, and I'd round him up and send him right over. Harry Hill was Dr. Hill, a young Epidemic Intelligence Service officer assigned to us from CDC. I remember Dr. Mollohan laughed. That would be fine, he said, but I didn't really need to bother. Because it just so happened that Dr. Harry Hill was sitting in his office that very minute. They had been talking about tick fever when Dr. Mollohan got his call from Atlanta. So Harry Hill came to the phone, and we talked for a couple of minutes. There wasn't a whole lot to say. He knew what to do. He was a trained epidemiologist. I simply told him to go ahead and do it."

Dr. Hill says: "It wasn't quite as simple as that. There was another matter of protocol. Before I could see the patient I had to go around to the Denver Department of Health and Hospitals and get permission. Children's Hospital is a municipal hospital. I picked up my wife — she had come down to Denver that morning with me — and I went through the necessary red tape. Then I was ready to begin. I found the intern assigned to the case, and we sat down together. He was shaken. He had just begun his training and Barbara Logan was his first patient. There can't be many doctors whose first case turned out to be plague. He showed me her chart and gave me what he had on her personal history. Then I saw Barbara. Her clinical picture was certainly compatible with a diagnosis of plague. 'Anybody could have made the diagnosis — if the possibility of plague had happened to enter his mind. But it hadn't. It very seldom does. Barbara was the third case of plague in Colorado in less than a year, and both of the others were also originally misdiagnosed. One was mistaken for streptococcal sore throat and the other for tularemia. But Barbara was lucky. Or maybe she was just naturally tough. Anyway, they got her started on the right drugs in time — on streptomycin and tetracycline instead of penicillin — and she survived. She made a full recovery. The others didn't. One of them died and the other ended up with permanent central-nervous-system damage.

"Barbara was too sick and too young for much of a talk, and I didn't stay with her long. I left the hospital and went out to the car, where my wife was waiting, and we drove back across town to the Logan house. Mrs. Logan was at home, and she was friendly and glad to help. What I hoped to get from her was some clue to the source of Barbara's infection. Sylvatic plague is hardly a common disease, but there have been enough cases over the years to establish a characteristic epidemiological pattern. The source, of course, is a wild rodent, and the setting is also wild. It's out in the wilderness

213

somewhere, a place where wild rodents abound. For example, that fatal Colorado case I mentioned was a boy on a ranch in Elbert County who shot and carried home a prairie dog. The other case was an oil-field worker in the mountains north of Grand Junction. The incubation period in plague is from two to six days. Barbara took sick on June 9. I naturally expected to hear from Mrs. Logan that there had been some sort of outing in the country soon after the first of June. But no. Barbara had hardly been off the block. She had been to City Park, only a few blocks away, on June 5, and two or three weeks before that, she had spent the day with an aunt on the east side of town, in Aurora, and that was all. If that was true — and how could I doubt it? — Barbara had been exposed to plague right here in the city of Denver.

"Which was crazy. Urban plague means rats. But Denver is unusual among American cities in that it has practically no rats. A continuing extermination program has just about wiped them out. However, I asked Mrs. Logan about rats. She said no. There weren't any rats, she said. There couldn't be any. An exterminator came to the house every week. I sat and thought a minute. There had to be an animal somewhere in the picture, I said. A sick or dead or dying animal. Mrs. Logan started to shake her head, and stopped. Did I say *dead* animals? Well, she didn't know, but she had heard that some dead squirrels had been found in the neighborhood. People had been finding dead squirrels off and on all spring. That was interesting. It was even promising. Fleas will desert a host soon after its death, but plague can be contracted from infected blood or saliva. I asked if Barbara was the kind of girl who might handle a dead animal. Indeed, she was, Mrs. Logan said. Very much so. She was a very inquisitive child. That was interesting, too. About these squirrels, I said — I supposed they were ground squirrels. What some people call chipmunks. Oh, no, Mrs. Logan said. They were regular squirrels. They were tree squirrels — like in the park.

"Well, I thanked Mrs. Logan and left. I didn't doubt there were tree squirrels around. The older parts of Denver are full of trees, and the Logan street was lined with big old elms. But I had always thought of plague as a disease of burrowing rodents. I went down to the car and started to get in, and saw some kids playing in the yard across the street. I told my wife I'd be right back. I went over to the kids and said I was an investigator and that I'd heard there were some dead squirrels around the neighborhood. Did they know anything about that? They all said 'Huh?' and 'What?,' and then one of them said sure — he knew where there was a dead squirrel. Did I want to see it? I said I certainly did, and he led me back around the house and out a gate and up an alley and over a fence and out another yard and across a street and around to another alley and stopped in front of a hollow tree. I looked in the hollow. I didn't have to see it — I could smell it. But there was enough of it left for laboratory examination. I went back to the car and told my wife about it and she looked sick, and we drove back to the hollow tree. There was an old fishing creel in the trunk of the car, and I scraped the remains of the squirrel or whatever it was into the creel and covered it up with an old blanket so it wouldn't smell too much. Then I looked around for a telephone and called Dr. Poland and told him what I'd found. He said OK, bring it in. He didn't sound too excited. My wife and I had dinner with a friend — and I remember how we all laughed when I said I had a squirrel with plague. Then we drove back to Fort

Collins. I stopped at the office and unloaded the squirrel or whatever it was and put it — creel and all — in a refrigerator in the lab, and left a note for Allan Barnes. Dr. Barnes is head of the mammalogy-entomology unit of the Zoonoses Section, and a very big man in plague. He'd take it on from there."

Dr. Barnes says: "It was a squirrel, all right — and a tree squirrel. It was the eastern fox squirrel, *Sciurus niger*. From the state of decomposition and an infestation of blowfly larvae, I judged it had been dead about a week. I handed the carcass over to Bruce Hudson in the laboratory to be tested for evidence of plague by his fluorescent-antibody staining technique. It was Dr. Hudson who adapted the FA test to plague. And a very good thing he did, too. The squirrel was far too dead to be tested by the standard bacteriological methods. I don't think I nourished any preconceived ideas. I felt pretty much the way Jack Poland felt. I wasn't too excited. I certainly didn't react the way I would have if Harry Hill had brought in a dead prairie dog. And I wasn't about to chase into Denver and start tearing down the Logan house looking for rats. I knew there were very few rats in Denver. I also knew that an eastern fox squirrel had been found dead of plague on the Stanford University campus back in 1966. It was an isolated case. The other campus squirrels tested out negative. But it was a case, a precedent. So I wasn't absolutely flabbergasted when Bruce Hudson walked in and told me that Harry Hill's specimen was positive for plague. It gave me a funny feeling, though. The Stanford case was a totally isolated case. This was different. We not only had a case of plague in an urban tree squirrel. We also had a case of human plague.

"Meanwhile, of course, I'd been talking with Jack Poland

and Harry Hill, and I had also been on the telephone to Denver. The people I mostly talked to there were Cecil Mollohan and Roy Cleere and Douglas McCluskie. Dr. Cleere is director of the Colorado State Department of Health, and Dr. McCluskie is director of the Division of Environmental Health for the city. The lab report was the push we needed, and we arranged for a meeting at Dr. Cleere's office on the afternoon of July 8. That was a Monday. I went down to Denver that morning and picked up Dr. McCluskie and we drove over to the Logan house. The Logan neighborhood, I should say. We weren't looking for Mrs. Logan. We were looking for more dead squirrels. There were kids playing on the block and women going marketing and old men just sitting around, and we talked to them all. Everybody seemed to know about the squirrels. One man told us he had found a dead squirrel in his yard as far back as May. He tossed it in his garbage can. And we found three dead squirrels. A man took us to one of them, and the kids showed us the others. They looked just as dead as Harry Hill's squirrel, but they weren't too decomposed to test.

"That sharpened the point of the meeting with Dr. Cleere and the others. One dead squirrel was simply one dead squirrel. But four dead squirrels was a die-off. And a die-off is always suspicious — whatever the cause of death. The other side of the picture, the human side, was fortunately unchanged. A check around the hospitals and clinics had been made, and there were no further cases of plague, or anything that even faintly looked like plague. There was still just Barbara Logan. Moreover, she would be discharged very shortly. The meeting drew up a report to inform physicians about her case and to alert them to the possibility of other victims. It reminded them of the clinical features of plague and pointed out the proper treatment. A general press release was also prepared. It gave the facts of Barbara's case, with a statement from Dr. Cleere to the effect that the situation was cause for concern but not for alarm, and it included a strong warning to the public against handling rodents, dead or alive. We also asked that any dead rodents be reported to the city health department. That about covers the meeting. Except that I was asked to head the field investigation. Dr. McCluskie and I sat down and made plans for a survey that would define the nature and the extent of the infection in the animal population. Denver has a great many tree squirrels. The eastern fox squirrel was introduced in 1908. By homesick Easterners, I suppose. Anyway, it prospered. There have also been immigrants. *S. niger* used to be strictly an eastern squirrel. You never saw it west of the Mississippi. But it's been slowly moving west across the plains — living off the wheatfields and nesting in the cottonwood river bottoms — since the late nineteen-twenties. Finally, a few years ago, it joined up with the others in Denver.

"We went to work the following day. The city had the collection facilities. Dr. McCluskie mobilized his Animal Control Division, and the dogcatchers picked up carcasses wherever we had a report, and turned them over to us for delivery to the laboratory for examination. Those dogcatchers really had to work. The dead-rodent reports rolled in — the phones rang all day long. Then the laboratory came through with a report on the carcasses Dr. McCluskie and I had found. They were plague-positive, too. So this wasn't anything like Stanford. This was a plague epizootic. Which brought up the crucial question of control. Control, in plague, means ectoparasite control, the eradication of the vector fleas. That was certainly all we wanted in this case. We didn't want to kill the Denver squirrels. But it was a tough nut to crack. We solved it with a system of baited stations rigged up in such a way that the squirrel got a harmless dusting of insecticide when he came onto the station. That took care of the fleas on his body, and also those back in his nest. We had some trouble with bait. Squirrels love peanut butter. But when we baited a station with peanut butter, the first squirrel to show up just settled down and ate and ate until the peanut butter was gone. We finally hit on pine cones impregnated with peanut butter. They carried those away. At the peak of our operation, we had eight hundred stations going.

"The active phase of the investigation lasted about three weeks. It began on July 9 and ran through the rest of the month. By the beginning of August, the peak of the epizootic had passed. We found our last positive on September 18. And Barbara Logan was still the only human case. The total tally was eight hundred and twenty-one carcasses collected and examined. Six hundred of them were tree squirrels. The others were other animals. None of those miscellaneous animals were positive for plague. Four hundred and ninety-three of the six hundred tree squirrels were found within the Denver city limits, the others on the outskirts. Only the Denver squirrels were plague positive. The positive squirrels totaled eighty-one. The curious thing was this. We had a big block map of the city set up in Dr. McCluskie's office and we kept a record with colored pins where every squirrel carcass was found. All but six of the positive squirrels were found in the northeast quadrant of Denver — the City Park area where Barbara lived. That would seem to be where the epizootic began and where it was somehow contained. There was also something else. The other thing was fleas. We collected a number of fleas. We found a few on newly dead squirrels and the rest we combed off about thirty live and healthy squirrels that we trapped for that purpose. The flea to which *S. niger* is normally host is *Orchopeas howardi*, and we found the expected number of them. But we also found three other kinds of fleas. We found a species that is normally found on ground squirrels, and we found two species that are normally found on rabbits. Let me say that the only infected fleas we found — the only plague-positive fleas — were a few *Orchopeas howardi*. The wild-rodent fleas were clean. Their mere presence, however, was bad news. I'm only thankful that it happened in a city like Denver — a city with practically no rats. Because a flea transfer like that very strongly suggests a wild-rodent intrusion into the urban environment. How this intrusion may have come about, I can't say. I don't know."

Neither does Dr. McCluskie. But he is willing to guess. He says: "I think what happened was this. I think some kid caught a ground squirrel up in the mountains and brought it home, and after a couple of days he got bored with it or his parents said get rid of it, and he let it out in City Park. I think it was just an accident like that. I hope so, anyway."

# The Dead Mosquitoes

Dr. John P. Conrad, Jr., a senior associate in a suburban pediatric group practice in Fresno, California, excused himself to the mother of the young patient in his consultation room and crossed the hall to take a telephone call in his office. The call was a request from a general practitioner on the other side of town named Robert Lanford to refer a patient to Dr. Conrad for immediate hospitalization and treatment. That morning — it was now around four o'clock in the afternoon (on October 4, 1961) — an eight-year-old boy whom I'll call Billy Cordoba had been brought to Dr. Lanford's office by his mother. Billy had been sent home sick from school. He was pale, his eyes had a glassy look, and his heart was a little fast. Dr. Lanford had examined him, found nothing significantly out of order, and sent him home to rest. But Billy was now back in his office, and there was no longer any doubt that he was sick. The manifestations of his illness now included a ghastlier pallor, a glassier look, a notably faster heart, rapid and irregular breathing, muscle twitches, diarrhea, nausea, vomiting, and abdominal pain. He was also confused in mind and almost comatose. Something about this inharmonious symphony of symptoms had prompted Dr. Lanford to make a urine-sugar test, and the results were strongly positive. That suggested a frightening possibility. He was afraid that Billy was a hitherto unsuspected diabetic on the brink of diabetic coma. In any event, he said, the boy was in urgent need of sophisticated help. Dr. Conrad agreed. He told Dr. Lanford that he shared his sense of urgency, and that he would arrange at once for Billy's admittance to Valley Children's Hospital.

Mrs. Cordoba drove her son to the hospital. Billy was admitted there at five o'clock. He was put to bed, and a sample of blood was taken for immediate laboratory analysis to confirm or deny the presence of diabetes. That had been ordered by Dr. Conrad when he made the admittance arrangements. When he himself reached the hospital, at a little before six, the results of the blood studies had been noted on Billy's chart. Dr. Conrad read them with a momentary lift of spirit. The relevant values (blood glucose, blood carbon dioxide, blood sodium, blood potassium, blood pH) were close enough to normal to make it comfortably certain that despite the earlier positive urinalysis the boy was not a diabetic. But that was all. Or practically all; the studies did show a morbid elevation in the white-blood-cell count. Other than that, the studies had no positive diagnostic significance. Dr. Conrad replaced the chart and went into Billy's room to take his first look at his patient. It was anything but reassuring. The boy was clearly sicker than he had been two hours before. Dr. Conrad sat down and began with care the standard physical examination. His findings were even more discordant than those recorded by Dr. Lanford. Billy's pulse was fast, his breathing was fast, his temperature was 100 degrees, his skin was pale and clammy, the pupils of his glassy eyes had shrunk to pinpoints, his face and arms were twitching, he was drooling saliva, and he appeared to be in almost constant abdominal pain. Twice during the short examination the pain was so great that he screamed. He was still confused, still comatose, still nauseated, still diarrheic. Dr. Conrad finished the examination and sorted out his impressions. They led in two distinctly different directions. One possibility was shigellosis, or bacillary dysentery. The other was chemical poisoning.

"I didn't particularly favor the idea of shigellosis," Dr. Conrad says. "It was simply suggested by some of the clinical evidence — the high white-cell count and the gastrointestinal symptoms. And I didn't favor it at all for very long. A shigella infection produces a rather distinctive kind of damage that can be detected by miscroscopic examination of a stool specimen. It isn't conclusive, but it's reliable enough to be useful. Well, I asked the laboratory for a report and the answer came back in a matter of minutes. Negative. I wasn't much surprised. Chemical poisoning had always been by far the stronger possibility. The very bizarreness of the symptoms was suggestive of poison. Certain particular symptoms were even more suggestive. Stupor. Abdominal pain. Salivation. But the real tipoff was those pinpoint pupils. What I had in mind was an insecticide — specifically, one containing an organic phosphate. That isn't as inspired as it may sound. Fresno County is a big agricultural county. It produces everything from cantaloupes

223

to cotton, and it uses tons of highly toxic chemicals. Including organic phosphates. Then Mrs. Cordoba said something that seemed to make my hunch a certainty. I was asking her the usual questions for Billy's personal history, and she remembered a remark that Billy made when he came home sick from school. The Cordobas live on the edge of town, and there are cultivated fields all around the stop where Billy waits for the bus. That morning, Billy said, there was a spray rig working in one of the fields and a spray plane flying back and forth overhead. Organic phosphates can enter the body in various ways, but the commonest route is absorption through the skin. Also, they work very fast. Symptoms can begin within a couple of hours of exposure. And it doesn't take much of the stuff to cause a lot of trouble. The fatal skin dose is only about five drops.

"I was practically certain that Billy had been poisoned by some organic-phosphate insecticide. I was sure enough to start treatment on that assumption. I followed the standard procedure. I ordered intravenous fluids to restore the loss of body fluids through sweating, salivation, and diarrhea, and a regimen of atropine — one milligram injected intramuscularly every two hours. Atropine is a lifesaving drug in organic-phosphate poisoning, because it relieves the threatening symptoms. It doesn't, however, get at the source. It doesn't eliminate the poison. The next step in the treatment involves a drug called PAM — pralidoxime chloride. But I couldn't take that step — not until I was absolutely certain. PAM is a little too specific to prescribe on mere suspicion. The definitive test for organic-phosphate poisoning is a blood test that measures the levels in the plasma and the red cells of an enzyme called cholinesterase. Cholinesterase is a kind of neural moderator. Its presence controls the accumulation of an ester that governs the transmission of impulses of the parasympathetic nervous system. Organic phosphates destroy cholinesterase, and the destruction of cholinesterase allows an excessive accumulation of the ester. The result is a powerful overstimulation of the parasympathetic nerves. The cholinesterase test is too elaborate for the average small hospital laboratory. The only laboratory equipped to do that kind of thing here is in the Poison Control Center at Fresno Community Hospital, down in the center of town. I drew a sample of blood and rounded up a messenger and got on the telephone to Dr. Bocian — Dr. J. J. Bocian, the director there. That was around seven o'clock. Dr. Bocian called me back around eight-thirty. He had the results of the test. Billy's plasma cholinesterase level was only forty percent of normal, and his red-cell level was a scant seventeen. His illness was definitely organic-phosphate poisoning.

"It was gratifying to know that I'd made a good guess. And that I'd been able to make it in time. But the really gratifying thing was Billy's response to atropine. By the time I had Dr. Bocian's definite diagnosis, Billy was just as definitely out of danger. His vital signs were all good. Moreover, he was beginning to look more alert. His pupils were coming back to normal size. And he wasn't salivating the way he had been. I was so satisfied that I decided to hold off on PAM. Atropine would continue to counteract the potentially dangerous neuromuscular symptoms, and time would do the rest. It would gradually bring the cholinesterase levels back to normal. I stayed at the hospital until about ten o'clock, and went home feeling pretty good. I had diagnosed the nature of Billy's illness, and he was responding well to treatment. And I thought I knew just how his illness had come about.

"But I was wrong about that. It wasn't the spray rig or the spray plane at the bus stop. It couldn't have been either of them. Mrs. Cordoba or her husband or somebody made some inquiries. Those rigs weren't spraying an organic phosphate. Or any kind of insecticide. The fields they were working were cotton fields, and they were spraying a defoliant to strip the plants for mechanical picking. But I wasn't mistaken about Billy. He continued to do just fine. I kept him on atropine and intravenous fluids for a total of forty-eight hours. His symptoms all subsided and his serum cholinesterase levels began to improve. At the end of the second hospital day, he showed a plasma level of forty-two percent of normal and a red-cell level of almost thirty-two. By the sixth day, the plasma level had risen to ninety-two percent of normal. The red-cell concentration is always slower to recover. It requires the formation of new cells. But it was up to forty percent. There was no reason to keep him in the hospital any longer. I could follow him the rest of the way as an out-patient. So I ordered his discharge."

Billy was discharged from Valley Children's Hospital to convalesce at home on October 9. That was a Monday. He remained at home, sleeping and eating and resting, until the following Monday, October 16. That afternoon, by prearrangement, Mrs. Cordoba drove him back across town to Dr. Conrad's office for what was expected to be a final physical examination and dismissal. Their appointment was for four o'clock, and they were on time.

"Billy looked fine," Dr. Conrad says. "And he was fine. Blood count, blood pressure, chest, pupils — everything was completely normal. So that was the happy ending of that. I walked Billy and his mother out to the waiting room and said goodbye and went back to my office and closed the case and rang for my next patient. I saw that patient and then the next, and then the receptionist called. She sounded almost frightened. Mrs. Cordoba was in the waiting room and she was practically hysterical. Billy was sick again. He was out in the car — too sick to even walk.

"It was true. I found Mrs. Cordoba and we went out to the car, and there he was, and he looked terrible. He looked shocky. His skin was cold and clammy with sweat, and he was salivating and breathing very fast, and he didn't seem to be able to move his legs. I didn't even go back in the building to say I was leaving. I just slid in beside Billy and told Mrs. Cordoba to head for the hospital. The hospital was only a block up the street, but on the way she told me what had happened. There wasn't much to tell. They had started home from my office, and they were almost there when all of a sudden Billy said he was sick. That was all she knew. She had turned around and driven right back to see me. But it was perfectly plain that this was the same thing all over again. Only worse — much worse. Dr. Bocian confirmed it later on in the evening. The serum cholinesterase levels were very low. The plasma level was down to twenty-seven percent of normal, and the red-cell level was only twenty. I got Billy started on atropine and intravenous fluids, but he didn't respond as he had before. Two hours after I got him into the hospital, he was seized with severe abdominal cramps and began to vomit. Then he developed diarrhea. It was time for PAM. I ordered an intravenous injection of five hundred milligrams. The next three hours were a little anxious, but then he began to improve. And the next morning he was very much better. He had had another five hundred milligrams of

PAM, and his cholinesterase levels were up enough to show that he was improving.

"That gave me a chance to think. Organic-phosphate poisoning is not a notifiable disease in California, so there had been no reason for me to report Billy's case to the Fresno County Public Health Department, but now I thought perhaps I should. I thought I had a lead that they might want to follow up. The lead was this: For a week at home, Billy had been as good as well. Then he got up and drove over here to my office, and less than an hour later he was critically ill again with organic-phosphate poisoning. I'm not an epidemiologist, but it seemed to me that the probable source of his exposure wasn't far to look for. It almost had to be either something in the family car or something he was wearing. When I got to my office on Wednesday morning, I called the Health Department and talked to Mary Hayes. Dr. Hayes has since left the Department but she was then the acting health officer, and she was very interested in my story. She said she would have somebody look into it. She called me back on Friday afternoon. They had the answer — or part of it, anyway. The source was Billy's clothes — his blue jeans. They were brand-new blue jeans that his mother had bought at a salvage store, and he had worn them only twice. He had worn them to school on the morning of October 4 and to my office on the afternoon of October 16. The Department had had the jeans tested and had found them contaminated with some form of organic phosphate.

"By that time, of course, Billy was recovering very nicely, and I could relax and begin to think about him as a case. It fascinated me. I'd never had a more dramatic experience in all my years of practice. Well, I'm on the staff at Fresno General

Hospital and I make teaching rounds there on Monday, Wednesday, and Friday mornings, and I was so fascinated by Billy and his poisoned blue jeans that I told the interns and residents about them on my next rounds. That was on Monday — Monday, October 23. The next day, I got a call from one of the residents, a doctor named Merritt C. Warren. He had a new patient on his service — an eight-year-old boy. We can call him Johnny Morales. Johnny had become sick at school that morning and had been admitted to the hospital by his family physician around noon. His initial symptoms were sweating, dizziness, and vomiting. He reached the hospital in a stumbling, mindless stupor. His pulse was fast, his respiration was weak and shallow, his face was contorted by muscular twitches, and the pupils of his eyes were contracted to pinpoints. He also had abdominal cramps. The family physician had tentatively diagnosed Johnny's trouble as acute rheumatic fever. Dr. Warren thought differently. He said he thought it was another case of poisoned pants. That was the way he put it. I thought he was probably right. And he was. Dr. Bocian confirmed it by a serum cholinesterase test a couple of hours later."

The inquiry by the Fresno County Public Health Department into the case of Billy Cordoba was conducted by an investigator in the Division of Environmental Health named R. E. Bergstrom. Mr. Bergstrom, who was then senior sanitarian in the Division (he is now its director), received the assignment within an hour of Dr. Conrad's report to Dr. Hayes on the morning of October 18. He and a colleague named Tiyo Yamaguchi were at the Cordoba house within an hour.

"We spent the rest of the day out there," Mr. Bergstrom says. "There and around the neighborhood. Mrs. Cordoba told us about the spraying operation near the bus stop. We followed that up and confirmed what she had learned herself. It was a standard cotton-defoliation spray — magnesium chloride and dinitrose. We went through the Cordoba house and the garage out back looking for anything in the way of a garden spray or insect bomb that might include an organic phosphate. Nothing. We examined the family car. Nothing. That left Billy's clothes, and Mrs. Cordoba showed us his blue jeans. She told us about them. They had been bought new about a month before at the salvage depot of the Valley Motor Lines. They were cheap, and she bought five pairs. But Billy had worn only one pair. And he had worn them only twice — to school that day and then to Dr. Conrad's office. I looked at Yamaguchi and he looked at me. We knew we had found what we were looking for. It had only to be proved. We wrapped up the jeans — all five pairs — for laboratory analysis. The Bureau of Vector Control of the California State Department of Public Health has a research station here, and we took the jeans over there the next morning. The first thing we wanted to know was whether they were contaminated. The Bureau had a quick and easy test for that. They breed mosquitoes at the station for experimental purposes, and they simply tossed the worn pair of jeans in with one of the colonies. I tell you, it was a sight to see. Those mosquitoes just curled up and died. It took only fifteen minutes. At the end of that time, every mosquito in the colony was dead. Not only that. There was another breeding colony about twenty feet away, and in about five more minutes all *those* mosquitoes were dead, too. The poison was that volatile.

"The next thing we wanted to know was the identity of the poison. We thought it was an organic phosphate, but was it? There is a color-reaction test that reveals the presence of phosphate. It takes a little longer than the mosquito test, but the Bureau had the chemistry to do it. We left the jeans with them to work on, and drove back in to town and down to the office of the Valley Motor Lines. It wasn't a very satisfactory visit. About all we learned was that there had been a sale of blue jeans at their salvage depot in September, and that all the jeans had been sold. They supposed the jeans had been damaged, but they didn't know in what way. They didn't know where the jeans had come from. They didn't know the number of jeans in the batch. All company records were stored at their main office, in Montebello, down in Los Angeles County. And, of course, they had no idea who had bought the jeans at the sale. We left them with the understanding that they would recover the relevant records. When we got back to the office, I called our friends at the Bureau of Vector Control. They were a lot more helpful. They had run the color-reaction test, and they had the result. It was positive for phosphate.

"That wasn't any great surprise, of course, but it was crucial. It established that Billy's blue jeans were in fact the source of his phosphate poisoning. All we needed to establish now was the source of the poison. And not just where it came from but also what it was. There are at least twenty-five commercial phosphate pesticides in common use. Like Parathion, for example. And Malathion. And Fenthion and Phosdrin and Diazinon and Dicapthon and Trithion and TEPP. And so on. So it might be easier to find out where it came from if we knew what particular phosphate pesticide we were looking for. Well, that kind of information can be got. It takes a little time, but it's possible by certain tests to identify an unknown phosphate pesticide. The Bureau couldn't do the analysis, but they knew who could — the Division of Chemistry of the California State Department of Agriculture, up in Sacramento. They said they would make the necessary arrangements. We should have a report in a week or ten days. The following day, we looked in at the Valley Motor Lines again. They still hadn't recovered the blue-jeans records. And the day after that it was the same. Apparently, it wasn't easy to get records out of Montebello. And then we heard about Johnny Morales. Dr. Conrad must have telephoned the news to Dr. Hayes. At any rate, we had the simple facts by the morning of October 25. We went over to the hospital — it's just across the street — and talked to Dr. Warren and to Mrs. Morales, and finally to Johnny himself. Johnny was still pitifully sick, but he had been treated in time with atropine and PAM, and he was off the critical list. His story was Billy Cordoba's story all over again. There was a new pair of blue jeans. They came, like Billy's, from the Valley Motor Lines' salvage depot. They carried the J. C. Penney label. So did Billy's. And, as we very soon found out, they were also heavily contaminated with an organic phosphate. Johnny had worn the jeans for the first time on October 20. He wore them to school that day and got sick around midmorning and was sent home. His mother put him to bed, and in a few days he was well. Then he put on his jeans again and went back to school, and ended up at Fresno General Hospital.

"Johnny's new jeans brought the total accounted for up to six. Mrs. Morales had bought only one pair. We still didn't know how many jeans had been sold in the sale, but it was certain that there were more than that. Dr. Hayes got in touch with all the local media. She called in the *Bee* and radio station KMJ and KMJ-TV, and it was all in the paper and on the air that evening, with a warning about the still unaccounted-for jeans and an appeal to the buyers to bring them in to the County Health Department for examination. The response was immediate, and good. As a matter of fact — although we didn't know it for a couple of weeks or more — it was one hundred percent. We received a total of ten pairs of J. C. Penney jeans, from six different buyers. They represented five families and an institution for children. We checked them out for recent illness and found four cases with much the same clinical picture. Four boys, in four of the five families. They were all recovered now, and they had all been differently diagnosed. Brain tumor was one diagnosis. Another was bulbar polio. One of the others was encephalitis. In retrospect, however, the signs and symptoms were unmistakably those of organic-phosphate poisoning, and when their jeans were tested, that confirmed it. But it was also a little peculiar. Not because they all recovered without specific treatment. That could be explained by light contamination or brief exposure, or both. The peculiar thing was that only those four got sick. What about the fifth family and the institution? They had each bought two pairs of jeans, and the jeans had been worn, but none of the boys who wore them had been even mildly ill. As I say, it seemed a little peculiar — until it turned out that those jeans were not contaminated. And the reason they were not contaminated was that they had been washed. And the reason nobody got sick was that they had been washed before they were worn. Billy and Johnny and the four other boys had worn their jeans the way most kids do. Just as they came from the store."

The transformation of Billy Cordoba's solitary seizure of organic-phosphate poisoning into a looming epidemic also changed the stature of the investigation. It was now imperative that the records of the Fresno blue-jeans sale be recovered from the Montebello office of the Valley Motor Lines, but doing so appeared to be beyond the strength of the Fresno County Public Health Department. Its exhortations did not carry across the state and into Los Angeles County. What was needed was the stronger voice of the California Department of Public Health. Accordingly, on October 26 Dr. Hayes invited that agency to take over the direction of the larger investigation, and her invitation was accepted. It was, however, immediately obvious to the Department of Public Health that in this instance the interrogational powers of a more specialized state agency would be even more compelling. That agency, whose assistance it sought and at once received, was the Public Utilities Commission, which at that time was charged with enforcing motor-carrier safety regulations.

The Public Utilities Commission's investigation was carried out by members of its Operations and Safety Section. They began their inquiry on October 27. Six days later — on Thursday, November 2 — they were pleased to receive from the Division of Chemistry of the Department of Agriculture (by way of the Bureau of Vector Control of the Department of Public Health) the ultimate test report on Billy Cordoba's blue jeans. It read, "The stained portion of the jeans contained Phosdrin, 4.8% by weight. The contaminant was specifically identified as Phosdrin by its characteristic infra-red absorption curve. . . ." This was useful information. They now were looking for a particular pesticide. That would make a difference in their progress through the labyrinth of bills of lading, manifests, and invoices. It remained only to link the contaminated J. C. Penney jeans in time and place with a quantity of Phosdrin.

They did so in just two weeks. The chain of circumstances that led to the poisoning of Billy Cordoba and the others had had its innocent beginning some eight months before at the Bayly Manufacturing Company, in the nearby town of Sanger. On February 3, 1961, a shipment of Bayly blue jeans — two large bales and a carton — consigned to a J. C. Penney store in Los Angeles was picked up at the Bayly plant by the Triangle Transfer Company, a Sanger trucking firm, and taken to the Fresno terminal of the Valley Motor Lines for transshipment south. Within an hour or two of its arrival in Fresno, the shipment was loaded aboard a Valley Lines trailer with a conglomeration of other freight. This freight consisted of machinery, machine parts, metal pumps, and a hundred twenty gallons of emulsifiable concentrate of Phosdrin, in one-gallon and five-gallon cans. The Phosdrin was the product of De Pester Western, Inc., a Fresno manufacturer, and was consigned to the Valley Chemical Company, at El Centro, down on the Mexican border.

The Valley Lines trailer left Fresno the following morning with this miscellaneous load, and that evening it reached the company terminal at Montebello, where the Phosdrin was unloaded for transshipment. Two days later, on February 6, it was put on board a truck operated by the Imperial Truck Lines, a Los Angeles firm, for the final leg of its journey. The Imperial driver made the usual precautionary inspection of his load before signing the delivery receipt, and found that one of the Phosdrin cans had sprung a leak. He traced the leak to a little puncture about three inches below the top of a five-gallon can. After some discussion, he signed the delivery receipt, but noted a formal exception to the shipment on the grounds that around a gallon of Phosdrin concentrate had been lost from the punctured can. (How the puncture occurred was never determined, but the loss was estimated in a subsequent claim by the Valley Chemical Company at one and one-eighth gallons, valued at twenty-four dollars and fifty cents.) Meanwhile, the shipment of blue jeans was delivered that same day by the original Valley Lines trailer to a J. C. Penney store in the Los Angeles suburb of Westchester. A shipping clerk there noticed a dark stain on the paper wrapping of one of the bales of jeans. He asked the driver about it, but the driver didn't know. He had never seen it before. The clerk went in and brought out the manager, and the manager told the Valley Lines driver that a damage claim would be filed if any of the jeans turned out to be soiled. Sixteen pairs of jeans were found to be stained with some unknown oily substance, and a claim for damages was filed on February 8. The claim was acknowledged by the Valley Motor Lines, and the sixteen pairs of jeans were stored in the J. C. Penney warehouse for pickup by the Valley Lines. They remained there all spring and all summer — until September 6. Then they were finally picked up and returned to Fresno. On September 19, they were put on cut-rate sale at the company's salvage-depot store. The jeans by then apparently looked all right. They might also by then have been as safe as they looked. It is possible. Seven months of storage in a warehouse subject to swings of heat and cold and damp and dry might well have caused much of the Phosdrin to volatilize and vanish. But the J. C. Penney warehouse was a new and modern warehouse. It was air-conditioned.

The Public Utilities Commission's report of these findings to the State Department of Public Health ended on a reassuring note. It concluded, "The staff's investigation of the personnel records and waybills of the two carriers involved failed to disclose any evidence of employee illnesses on the days in question or subsequent thereto, and failed to disclose any evidence that foodstuffs or other personal effects, including clothing, had been contaminated."

The Commission's report was not, however, the end of its interest in the matter. It at once instituted an investigation into the general operations, safety practices, equipment, and facilities of the Valley Motor Lines and the Imperial Truck Lines, and on February 14, 1962, a public hearing on the results of that investigation was held at Fresno. Both companies were found guilty of carelessness, and admonished and fined. The Valley Lines was fined five thousand dollars — the maximum penalty — and the Imperial Lines was fined twenty-five hundred dollars.

# The Case
# of Mrs. Carter

The case of the woman whom I'll call Linda Mae Carter — Mrs. Joseph Carter — first came to the attention of Dr. Louis Cohen, an internist in Topeka, Kansas, on the morning of February 24, 1962. It was brought to his attention by a colleague on the staff of the Topeka State Hospital. Mrs. Carter, his colleague told him over the telephone, was thirty-three years old and the wife of a skilled machinist. The Carters had one child, a boy of three. Mrs. Carter had been a patient at Topeka State for almost three months. She had been admitted on November 29 for evaluation of a progressive disabling disease tentatively diagnosed as amyotrophic lateral sclerosis. She was further disabled by two hip fractures that had failed to mend properly, and by a severe mental depression. The hospital was discharging her that afternoon. There had been no improvement in her physical condition, and a recent psychiatric diagnosis had described her as a hysterical personality with neurotic or psychotic potentialities, but the hospital felt that she would be more comfortable at home with her family. Continued hospitalization seemed useless, and might even be damaging to so young a woman. The only trouble was that the Carters had no regular physician. Might he refer Mrs. Carter and her husband to Dr. Cohen? Dr. Cohen hesitated. It sounded like a discouraging case, but he couldn't very well say no. He told him to go ahead.

"That was a Saturday," Dr. Cohen says. "I heard from the Carters on Monday. I called my office from the hospital — Stormont-Vail Hospital — as I always do after my morning rounds, and my nurse gave me the morning calls and messages. One of the calls was from Joseph Carter. His wife wanted to see me — sometime that day, if possible. Well, right then was as good a time as any, so I asked my nurse to call and say I'd be over directly. I got there around ten o'clock. It was a fairly new house on an unpaved road in a kind of development way out on the north side of town. Carter was at work by then, and a neighbor girl opened the door. They had got her in as a combination nurse and babysitter. She took me into the bedroom. Mrs. Carter was lying there flat on her back in a hospital bed. She was a nice-looking woman with pretty black hair, but her face was as white as a sheet, and she was nothing but skin and bones.

"I introduced myself and sat down by the bed, and we talked for a couple of minutes. Mrs. Carter had no particular reason for calling me. I mean, nothing new had happened since Saturday — since she left the hospital. She simply wanted to meet me, and she hoped I could do something to help her.

Nobody else had been able to, she said. I said I'd do the best I could. We talked a little more, and then I examined her. It was pathetic. She was really disabled. She was doubly disabled. She was flat on her back because of her fractured hips, but that was only part of it. She was also immobilized by a permanent contraction of the muscles of her legs and abdomen. Her body was pulled as taut as a bowstring. And not only that. Every now and then, she told me, her muscles would suddenly pull even tighter, and she would go into a spasm. I knew what she meant, and I could imagine how it must have felt. It would have been a seizure like the spasms in tetanus or in strychnine poisoning. A powerful convulsion. Those symptoms — the stiffness and the spasms — were manifestations, of course, of the disease that was thought to be amyotrophic lateral sclerosis. Amyotrophic lateral sclerosis is a degenerative disease of the central nervous system. It's somewhat on the order of multiple sclerosis — what they used to call 'Lou Gehrig disease.' Well, I examined her as carefully as I could in the circumstances, and I must say I wasn't particularly impressed by the amyotrophic-lateral-sclerosis hypothesis. One of the usual manifestations of that disease is muscle fasciculations. That's a spontaneous muscular quivering. It's like the deliberate twitch that a horse gives when he wants to shake off a fly. Another, though less frequent, manifestation is a positive Babinski reflex. Babinski's reflex is an upturning of the big toe when the sole of the foot is stroked. A turned-up toe is an indication of damage to the pyramidal tract of the brain and spinal cord. Also, there is usually some spasticity in the lower legs. But Mrs. Carter had a negative, or normal, Babinski, and I found no suggestion of either muscle fasciculations or spasticity.

"So I had my doubts about amyotrophic lateral sclerosis. And yet I couldn't absolutely rule it out. The only certainty was that I needed to know a great deal more about this case than I did. Even the general nature of Mrs. Carter's trouble was not entirely clear. She seemed to be the victim of some central-nervous-system disease, but maybe not. Maybe that was only the way it looked. I remembered that the State Hospital had described her as a hysterical personality. I didn't find her very stable myself. Actually, she was rather hostile. She was more or less hostile all the time I was with her. Still, we talked. We talked about her illness. And the more we talked, the less her hostility bothered me. By the time I left, it hardly bothered me at all. I could understand why she acted that way. I mean, I had an inkling. It wasn't until I dug into her medical history and saw just what she'd been through that I really understood."

Mrs. Carter's trouble began in 1959. One day in early August of that year, she stumbled and fell while getting out of the family car. She wasn't hurt, but the accident unnerved her. It was her conviction that it hadn't been an ordinary accident. There was something wrong with her legs. They had a funny feeling. This impression persisted, and as summer ended and autumn came on she identified the feeling as a stiffness. It was a sudden tightening of the leg muscles, and it seemed to occur at moments of emotional stress. Mrs. Carter had a job at that time as a clerk in a Topeka business office, and she became aware that any little excitement — a teasing remark by one of her fellow-workers — might bring on a stiffening contraction. The spasms lasted for several minutes, and while they lasted her legs were locked at the knee. She could walk only with a painful stiff-legged lurch. Around Thanksgiving, the spasms became more frequent. They also lasted longer, and it seemed to take less and less to bring them on. The telephone, the doorbell, a shout — any unexpected noise would throw her into a spasm, and she found that she was especially susceptible just before a menstrual period. Even a sudden quickening of pace would often excite a seizure. She developed a frantic fear of falling, and refused to ride on escalators or to go through revolving doors. She began to cry at the slightest provocation. Shortly after Christmas — in January of 1960 — she called a physician recommended by a friend, and made an appointment for a consultation.

The physician Mrs. Carter consulted was an internist whom I'll call Dr. Warren. He asked her the usual questions and then performed the usual comprehensive examination. The results of the examination were unequivocally normal. There was no evidence of any fundamental physical derangement. It was equally clear, however, that Mrs. Carter was physically disabled. Dr. Warren resolved this perplexity in the standard modern manner. It was his impression, he told Mrs. Carter, that her trouble was functional rather than constitutional in origin. A psychiatric examination was therefore indicated. If Mrs. Carter wished, he would be glad to refer her to a psychiatrist in whom he had every confidence. Mrs. Carter thanked him, took the name of the recommended psychiatrist, and went home.

Mrs. Carter considered calling Dr. Warren's psychiatrist. She discussed the matter with her husband and thought about it for several days. She wanted to call, and yet she didn't. The idea of a psychiatric examination was somehow very disturbing. The days, the weeks, the months went by, and she never made the call. Instead, toward the end of July she telephoned Dr. Warren again and made another appointment. The reason for the consultation was a new set of muscular symptoms. In addition to the spasms that locked her knees, she now had begun to suffer from similar spasms in the muscles of her neck. The muscles there were tender, and they often ached. So did those in her shoulders. Dr. Warren examined her again. The examination confirmed her new complaints. It also further confirmed his impression that her symptoms were psychogenic. He gave her a prescription for phenobarbital to ease her nervousness, and urged her once more to consult his psychiatric colleague. Mrs. Carter said she would.

But she didn't. Nor did she call on Dr. Warren again. With the help of phenobarbital, she continued on her own for three months longer. Then, in November, she consulted another friend and telephoned another physician. I'll call him Dr. Rushing. His impression of Mrs. Carter and of the nature of her illness was much the same as that affirmed and reaffirmed by Dr. Warren. He, too, concluded that what she needed was psychiatric treatment. However, before passing her along to psychiatry, he thought it might be prudent to arrange for a neurological consultation. Mrs. Carter had no objection to that, and a few days later she was admitted for observation to Stormont-Vail Hospital. The observing neurologist returned her to Dr. Rushing with a report that entirely confirmed the latter's understanding of the matter. There was no evidence of any neurological disease — no aberrant reflexes, no abnormal modalities of sensation, no synaptic ambiguities. On the other hand, the neurologist added, there was abundant evidence of "emotional illness . . . lying somewhere in the neurotic range, with components of anxiety, hysteria, and the possibility of a little depression." Psychiatric evaluation was strongly recommended.

Dr. Rushing conferred with Mrs. Carter the following week, and he succeeded where Dr. Warren had failed. Mrs. Carter agreed to let him refer her to the municipal Family Service and Guidance Center of Topeka for psychiatric examination and counseling. Her name was put on the waiting list there, and when the Center called her, early in January of 1961, she responded to the call. The results of the examination were a gratifying justification of the neurologist's apprehension and the suspicions of Dr. Warren and Dr. Rushing. Mrs. Carter was emotionally ill, and the specific character of her illness was diagnosed as a "conversion reaction, or schizophrenic reaction, schizo-affective-type." She was instructed to return to the Center for a psychotherapeutic consultation. She returned for two or three consultations with a designated staff psychiatrist, and then — losing interest or patience or confidence — dropped out of the course. A week or two later, around the middle of March, she called another psychiatrist, a man in private practice, and arranged for an office consultation. Her physical condition by then had conspicuously worsened. The psychiatrist noted that she arrived on the arm of her husband, and was unable to walk across the room without help. He also noted that she "kept her handkerchief over her face at all times" and that her general behavior was "inappropriate." She was, in addition, "quite uncooperative." At the end of the consultation, Mrs. Carter asked for a prescription for phenobarbital. The psychiatrist, detecting in her manner a hint of possible dependence, refused. Instead, he gave her a prescription for mephenesin, a muscle relaxant and a non-addictive drug, and urged her to resume her consultations at the Family Service and Guidance Center. But nothing came of either remedy. Mrs. Carter ignored his advice, and the mephenesin failed to control the crippling muscle spasms. The spasms spread from her legs to her thighs and upward to her abdomen, and the seizures became more violent and more frequent. Early in April, she found it necessary to resign her job. She was practically immobilized by almost daily seizures.

The accident in which Mrs. Carter suffered the first of her two hip fractures occurred on June 21. That morning, as usual, she awakened early, at about six-thirty, and, as usual, asked her husband to help her out of bed. His help had become essential. Her muscles were now so tightly drawn that she couldn't bend at either the waist or the knees. Carter picked her up like a log, swung her gently around, and lowered her feet to the floor. Her heels found a purchase and he raised her stiffly erect. Her body gave a sudden spastic wrench. There was a crack like the sound of a snapping twig, and Mrs. Carter screamed. Carter stood transfixed. Mrs. Carter screamed again, and then began to moan. Carter laid her back on the bed and ran to the telephone and called the Topeka ambulance service. Mrs. Carter was carried into the emergency room of Stormont-Vail Hospital at about seven-thirty. An X-ray examination revealed an intracapsular fracture of the left hip. The bone was set, and fixed in place with a flanged, triangular five-inch length of stainless steel known to surgery as a Smith-Petersen nail. Mrs. Carter remained in the hospital for almost two weeks. Her hip appeared to be mending normally, and on July 4 she was discharged to convalesce at home.

Mrs. Carter spent the summer on her back in bed. The muscle spasms and the spells of crying continued. Her emotions were stretched as tight as her leg and abdominal muscles, and they were equally sensitive to even the slightest jar. She was still confined to bed when the accident in which she suffered her second hip fracture occurred. That was on October 14, around seven o'clock in the morning. Mrs. Carter had awakened that morning with a soreness at the base of her spine that radiated into her right hip. She asked her husband to massage it. She had experienced this soreness several times before and had found that a gentle massage would relieve it. Mrs. Carter lay on her back, and her husband kneaded her hip and upper thigh. After two or three minutes, she asked him to massage her spine, and moved to turn on her stomach. Her body arched in a spasm — and Carter again heard a crack like the sound of a snapping twig. Mrs. Carter screamed.

An X-ray examination at Stormont-Vail Hospital, to which Mrs. Carter was again conveyed by ambulance, revealed an intracapsular fracture of the right hip. It also revealed that her fractured left hip was unhealed. The Smith-Petersen nail had not been strong enough to withstand the wrench of almost daily muscle spasms, and the bone ends had gradually pulled apart. The attending surgeon had planned to fix the new fracture with another Smith-Petersen nail, but the evidence of the second X-ray immediately changed his mind. He used instead a system of Hague pins. A Hague pin is a stainless-steel bolt with threads at one end to receive a securing nut. The pins chosen by Mrs. Carter's surgeon were about six inches long and just over an eighth of an inch in diameter. He fixed the right hip fracture with three Hague pins, and then removed the loosened nail from the other hip and replaced it with a bone graft and another set of three pins. It was during Mrs. Carter's convalescence from that double operation that a tentative diagnosis of amyotrophic lateral sclerosis was offered as a possible supplement to the continuing psychiatric evaluation. Mrs. Carter remained at Stormont-Vail until November 29. That was when she was admitted to Topeka State Hospital. A few weeks after her arrival there, she suffered a series of spasms so violent that her fractures were again undone. The spasms were, in fact, so violent that they bent the six Hague pins. The pins still held, but the damage now was irreparable. A normal union of her broken bones could never be achieved as long as her spasms continued, and Mrs. Carter was all but completely helpless.

It took Dr. Cohen several days to root out and review Mrs. Carter's medical history. His findings left him sympathetic but confused. In a memorandum he made at the time, he noted, "Fantastic as it may seem, the possibility must be considered that this patient has fractured both hips during violent muscle spasms of psychic origin. Metabolic bone disease must be considered, and appropriate studies are recommended to rule out this factor. Although the history is against this, a convulsive disorder must be ruled out. Repeat neurological evaluation is thus suggested." Dr. Cohen contemplated this brier patch of diagnostic contradictions, and then, with more hope than expectation, arranged with his colleague at Topeka State Hospital for a thorough reevaluation of the neurological evidence in their file on Mrs. Carter. Meanwhile, he did what he could to make her less uncomfortable. The means he finally settled on was a muscle-relaxant drug known to pharmacology as chlorzoxazone. Its impact, though slight, was perceptible. Chlorzoxazone (in doses of five hundred milligrams three times a day) had no effect on the shackling muscular rigidity, but it somewhat tempered the ferocity of the periodic spasms. That was a small but not insignificant blessing.

A report on the Topeka State review of Mrs. Carter's case reached Dr. Cohen on May 10. It took the form of a letter from his colleague on the hospital staff and (in its essentials) read, "We had an interesting panel discussion. . . . The neurology consultants were unable to make a diagnosis accounting for all the clinical symptoms and signs. There are many features about the patient that did not fit within the frame of the so-called amyotrophic lateral sclerosis group. The patient did not show any atrophy of muscles or muscle fasciculations, and apparently did not suffer from anterior horn [of the spinal cord] degeneration. The hip fractures did not show any degree of healing. The osteoporosis of both hips was still observed. . . . An electromyogram [a recorded depiction of muscular contraction] was normal. Serum sodium, potassium chloride, calcium phosphorous, alkaline phosphatase and acid phosphatase, BUN, Creatinine, uric acid, LDH, LAP, blood sugar, SGOT, SGPT, and CRP were all within limits of normal." Dr. Cohen read the report without elation. Its value was almost entirely negative. Osteoporosis, the one pathological finding, is an abnormal porosity, or rarefaction, of the bones. Bones thus weakened may sometimes fracture spontaneously. There was, however, no reason to believe that osteoporosis was a significant factor in Mrs. Carter's hip fractures. Her fractures were spontaneous fractures, but it was an aberrant force of muscle, rather than a weakness of bone, that brought them about.

Dr. Cohen added the Topeka State report to his file on Mrs. Carter and resumed his diagnostic search. It now took him exclusively to the library. In spite of the lack of neurological evidence, he was increasingly inclined to feel that Mrs. Carter's trouble was basically neurological, and the literature he searched was largely in the field of neuromuscular disorders. His explorations led him through many clinical journals and through the ranks of many clinical investigators, and among those many investigators the name of one turned up so often that it fixed itself in his mind. This was a member of the neurology section of the Mayo Clinic named Donald W. Mulder. There was nothing relevantly revelatory in the writings of Dr. Mulder that came to Dr. Cohen's attention, but they had a decisive impact. He emerged one evening from a Mulder paper with both a sense of resignation and a sudden flash of hope. He faced and accepted the probability that an accurate diagnosis of Mrs. Carter's trouble was beyond him. It might not, however, be beyond the reach of Dr. Mulder.

Mrs. Carter and her husband knew the Mayo Clinic by reputation, and since its reputation is an inspiring one, they responded to Dr. Cohen's proposal with an almost euphoric approval. The only problem was Mrs. Carter's total immobility, but Mr. Carter provided an answer to that. They could make the trip by trailer. Rochester, Minnesota, the seat of the Mayo Clinic, was not much more than five hundred miles from Topeka.

On June 5, Dr. Cohen sat down and wrote an introductory letter to Dr. Mulder. He had, he said, a "very interesting" patient whom he would like to refer for diagnosis and possible suggestions for treatment. He then related her appalling history — the devastating muscular contractions, the pathological hip fractures, the contradictory diagnoses — and described the treatment she was now receiving. It was his feeling, he went on to say, that she might have an aneurysm pressing on the pyramidal tract of the spinal cord, or a "space-occupying lesion." He ended his letter with a warning that Mrs. Carter "would have to be admitted directly to the hospital" and that she would arrive by trailer.

Dr. Mulder's reply was prompt and eagerly affirmative. It was also brief and to the point. Dr. Mulder was looking forward to seeing "this very interesting patient," and arrangements were being made for her admission to the neurology service at the Methodist-Worrall Hospital, in Rochester, on Monday, June 11. He would keep Dr. Cohen informed of Mrs. Carter's progress.

The Carters reached Rochester on June 10, and Mrs. Carter was admitted to the hospital the following morning. She remained there under observation and examination until July 3. On July 14, Dr. Mulder's progress report came through, and it was indeed a report of progress. It introduced Dr. Cohen to a disease of which he had never heard, and to a drug so new that it was not yet on the market.

Dr. Mulder began with an expression of thanks for the opportunity of seeing Mrs. Carter in neurological consultation. He and his colleagues were very much interested in her problem. It was provocatively reminiscent. Nevertheless, the possibility that she might be suffering from a spinal-cord tumor or spinal-cord lesion "with secondary muscle spasm" was routinely considered. The indicated tests — an X-ray examination of the muscle tissue, an X-ray examination of the spinal cord, and an examination of the spinal fluid — were made. The results, however, were all essentially normal. That returned them to their first impression. It was their conclusion that Mrs. Carter's clinical syndrome might best be classified as being the "stiff-man syndrome." This syndrome had recently been found to respond to a new drug called Valium, and Mrs. Carter had been so treated and with apparent success. He would see that Dr. Cohen received a supply of the drug. He wished Dr. Cohen and Mrs. Carter well, and hoped to be kept informed of the latter's progress.

Dr. Cohen's decision to solicit help for Mrs. Carter at the Mayo Clinic was more than just a happy one. It was providential as well. The Mayo Clinic was then the only medical center in the world where the stiff-man syndrome could be both readily diagnosed and efficaciously treated. Few physicians even now have ever heard of it. The syndrome is known at the Mayo Clinic because it was there that it was first recognized as an entity. It also was first successfully treated there, and it was named by Mayo investigators.

Its discoverers were two Mayo neurologists — Frederick P. Moersch and Henry W. Woltman. They announced their discovery in a report to the *Proceedings of the Staff Meetings of the Mayo Clinic*, entitled "Progressive Fluctuating Muscular Rigidity and Spasm ('Stiff-Man' Syndrome): Report of a Case and Some Observations in Thirteen Other Cases," in 1956. It was not a hasty announcement. The report began, "In the summer of 1924, an Iowa farmer, aged 49 years, came to the Clinic because of 'muscle stiffness and difficulty in walking.'" It continued:

His disability . . . had begun insidiously in 1920 with episodes of tightening of the muscles of his neck. Gradually, these attacks had increased in frequency, in severity, and in duration. The tightening had spread to include the muscles of the shoulders and upper portion of the back. In March of 1923, after a fall, which had appeared to have no serious consequences other than to confine the man to bed for a few days, his muscular condition had worsened. His neck muscles had remained rigid most of the time, and his head could be brought forward only with great effort. Also, the abdominal muscles and, to a lesser degree, those of the lower part of the back and those of the thighs had partaken of this same stiffness or tightness. Moreover, the rigidity had been punctuated by intermittent and moderately painful spasms. As might be expected, this behavior of his muscles had interfered with walking. His gait had become slow and awkward and, when spasms had supervened, he might "fall as a wooden man." He had observed that noise, a sudden jar, or voluntary movement often precipitated these spasms. To arise from a seated position he frequently required assistance. . . . Nothing helpful to diagnosis was learned from routine physical [and] neurologic examination. . . . We could not make a diagnosis, but the unusual condition interested us no end and, to associate it with a memorable and descriptive term that could not be taken by anyone to be final, we nicknamed it the "stiff-man syndrome." In the absence of a diagnosis, and without knowledge of specific treatment, we observed the effects of bromides, of intramuscular administration of magnesium sulfate, and of sedation with barbiturates, but these helped only temporarily. . . . We were not privileged to examine this patient again. . . . He reported last in 1932. . . . He could be on his feet, but he was weak and could take only a few steps unassisted.

This ends our account of that case, but the clinical picture so imprinted itself on our minds that in the course of the following years we recognized the same syndrome in . . . thirteen other cases.

The records of these fourteen cases were similar. There was some variation in rapidity of onset, in degree and extent of muscular rigidity, and in associated spasms. Some patients complained slightly of pain that occurred with the spasms, and in four instances pain was of major importance. A critical review of the records suggested no common cause. . . . Of our fourteen patients, ten were males and four were females. The age of onset of the illness varied from twenty-eight to fifty-four years. . . . It is worth noting that the malady frequently was considered to be functional, especially in its early stages. Of our fourteen patients, four came to us without previous diagnosis. In five cases, a diagnosis of "functional condition" had been made by the referring physicians, and one of these patients had been given several electric-shock treatments to no avail. We, too, considered the possibility of a functional disorder in these five cases, and in several we pursued psychotherapy, including hypnosis in one case, before realizing our error. The previous diagnosis made in the remaining five cases was chronic tetany [a convulsive muscular disorder of metabolic origin] in two, and, respectively, dystonia [a disturbance in muscular tonicity], stroke, and arthritis in three. . . . In six cases the muscles of the trunk were first affected, in four cases the muscles of the neck and shoulders, and in the remaining four, the muscles of the limbs. Of these latter four cases, the legs were first involved in three, and a leg and the ipsilateral arm in the fourth. In all instances, the affliction spread to include other muscles. . . . Routine physical examination of the patients did not help toward diagnosis. Neurologic examination of the patients demonstrated only fluctuating muscular rigidity and spasm. . . .

Thus our story ceases for the present. The threads are there but, in spite of their being woven into a fairly constant pattern, the completed design awaits added study. Whether the rigidity occurred reflexly by way of the spinal cord, or whether it represented involvement of the basal ganglia, we could not decide. . . . Because of the fluctuating intensity of symptoms and because four patients had reducing substances in the urine, a metabolic basis for the malady should be considered.

The completed design of the stiff-man syndrome still awaits added study. It is generally accepted that the disease has its seat in the spinal cord, and that both the creeping rigidity and the volcanic spasms are brought about (like the convulsions in strychnine poisoning and in tetanus) by a disturbance in the polarizing elements called synapses, which separate one cell from another in the neuron chains along which nervous impulses travel. This disturbance, it is thought, manifests itself as a suppression of synaptic inhibition, and a kind of neuromuscular anarchy results. The nature of that fundamental disturbance, however, remains a total mystery. The years since the publication of "Progressive Fluctuating Muscular Rigidity and Spasm" have produced just two real certainties about the stiff-man syndrome. One of these, the discovery of a Mayo Clinic neurologist named Frank M. Howard, is that a drug variously known as diazepam, Valium, and 7-chloro-1, 3-dihydro-1-methyl-5-phenyl-2H-1, 4-benzodiazepin-2-one has the power to throttle its symptoms. The other is that the stiff-man syndrome is not a phenomenon peculiar to the American Middle West. Clinicians have reported cases in other parts of this country and in Britain, Germany, and Spain. In the spring of 1962, when Mrs. Carter made her instructive visit to the Mayo Clinic, the number of cases of stiff-man syndrome on record was twenty-three. She brought the total up to twenty-four.

Dr. Cohen was out of town when Mrs. Carter returned from the Mayo Clinic. He didn't see her until the day he received Dr. Mulder's revelatory letter. Mrs. Carter was another revelation. Her response to diazepam had been complete. The muscle spasms had ceased, and her leg and abdominal muscles were normally relaxed. Moreover, for the first time in almost three years she was able to make herself comfortable.

"Not only physically comfortable," Dr. Cohen says. "She also seemed to be more comfortable in her mind. She was beginning to stop just lying there and waiting for the next spasm to hit. She was beginning to hope. And so was I. With those terrible spasms under real control, her fractures would finally have a chance to mend. She would probably always be a cripple. That was almost certain. But she might someday be able to walk a little. It all depended on diazepam. The only trouble was that diazepam wasn't on the market yet. It didn't become generally available in this part of the country until about 1964. Mrs. Carter had a supply on hand. Dr. Mulder had fixed the dosage at fifteen milligrams four times a day, and he had given her enough tablets to last for three or four weeks. After that, it was up to me. I wrote to the people who made it — the pharmaceutical firm of Hoffmann-La Roche, in Nutley, New Jersey — and they wrote right back. They were very much interested in the case I described, and they would be glad to provide me with a regular supply of Valium — that's their brand name for diazepam — for experimental clinical use.

"Which they did. They worked out the amount I needed, and every month or so they sent me something like five hundred five-milligram tablets, and I rationed them out to Mrs. Carter. I followed the dosage set by Dr. Mulder. It was fairly heavy. Sixty milligrams a day is a lot of diazepam. But it takes that much to do the job in the stiff-man syndrome. And it did a wonderful job. Mrs. Carter continued to respond. Her hips began to knit, and in less than a year she was up and walking with the help of a walker. Her progress was all I had hoped for. There was only one incident — one interruption. That one was plenty, though. I don't know if you've ever seen a Valium label, or one of the ads for Valium. There's a paragraph there headed 'Side Effects.' The last sentence reads, 'Abrupt cessation after prolonged overdosage may produce withdrawal symptoms similar to those seen with barbiturates, meprobamate, and chlordiazepoxide HCl.' The reason for that paragraph is a number of experiences very much like mine. And mine was one of the scares of my life.

"It happened in the second year of treatment, in December 1963. I don't know how it happened — and it doesn't matter. But there was a slipup here or there or somewhere, and we ran out of diazepam. I sent an airmail letter off to Hoffmann-La Roche, but I wasn't particularly worried. I didn't think that a couple of days off diazepam would seriously revive her symptoms. And they didn't. She seemed to be all right — for a day or two. She was much the same as ever. She then began to act a little anxious, and there was some tremor and twitching. I still wasn't really worried — only a bit uneasy. Then, all of a sudden, I got a call from Mr. Carter. His wife was having convulsions. For a moment, I thought he meant a return of the stiff-man spasms. But it wasn't that. I realized a moment later that he was describing a status-epilepticus seizure, and I told him I'd get out there as fast as I could. Status epilepticus is a series of epileptic-like seizures, and it represents a real medical emergency. The seizures often come so fast the patient has no chance to breathe. There are several drugs that are more or less effective in controlling status epilepticus. The drug I used was sodium pentobarbital. It worked well enough. Then I called an ambulance and got her to the hospital. She had no more seizures that day or that night, and the next morning a new supply of diazepam arrived by special-delivery airmail.

"So it turned out to be just an incident. The effect of diazepam is practically immediate. There was no harm done. There was no setback. There were no aftereffects. Mrs. Carter continued to improve. In a few more months, she could walk around the room by holding on to the furniture. Then she was doing the cooking again, and even a little house-work. And then she got to the point where she could walk just leaning on her husband's arm. They even go out now and then. The last time I saw her, she was talking about getting a job."

# Something
# a Little Unusual

Around noon on October 28, 1963, five people — two men, two women, and a child — sat down to midday dinner in the kitchen of a house they shared on a tobacco farm in the Caney Valley hills of Hawkins County, Tennessee, about fifteen miles southwest of Kingsport. They were (I'll say) Homer Mason and his wife, Louise; the latter's sister and her husband, Grace and Leroy Smart; and the Smarts' son, a boy of three called Buddy. Mason and the two women had spent the morning in the barn stripping and bundling cured tobacco leaves for the market. Smart had had other work to do, and it was he who prepared the meal. It consisted of split-pea soup, spaghetti with meat sauce, sliced tomatoes, sweet milk, and corn bread. Mason was the first to finish eating. He told his wife and Mrs. Smart that he would meet them down at the barn. He was going to stop by the cowshed for a look at an ailing calf. He left the house and crossed the yard, and suddenly began to stagger. He lurched against a tree. The barnyard tilted and the sky reeled. For a moment, Mason clung to the tree, and then it, too, began to sway. He turned and staggered back across the pitching barnyard toward the house. He stopped and blinked and shook his head. Something was happening to his eyes. The house was hardly fifty yards away, but he could only just make it out. He seemed to be going blind.

So did Mrs. Smart. When Mason stumbled into the kitchen, she was sitting there at the table with her head in her hands and moaning. Her husband stood beside her. Mrs. Mason stood on the other side of the table with Buddy in her arms. He was staring at his mother and whimpering. Mason dropped into a chair, and Mrs. Smart raised her head. "Homer, I can't hardly see," she said. "I think I'm going blind."

"Me, too," Mason said.

"And I'm dizzy," she said. "I tried to stand up a few minutes ago and everything was just spinning. I felt like a drunk man."

"She like to fell," Smart said. "I had to catch her."

"Same here," Mason said. "I feel the same way."

"Then it isn't just me," Mrs. Smart said. "I thought it was just me. Because Leroy feels all right, and so do Louise and Buddy."

"You'll be all right, honey," Smart said. "Everything's going to be all right."

"I don't feel as good as I did," Mrs. Mason said, and abruptly sat down. "There's something funny in my head. I feel kind of goofy."

Mrs. Smart gave a little wail. "Oh, my gosh!" she said. "I even feel sick to my stomach! What is it, Homer? What's the matter?"

"I don't know," Mason said. "Maybe we've been poisoned. There's three of us don't feel right — you and me and Louise. And there was only just the three of us working down in the barn this morning." He stopped and licked his lips. They felt stiff and cracked, and his mouth was dry. "Maybe we've got tobacco poisoning," he said. "We've all of us got the nicotine stain on our hands. Some of it maybe come off in our food."

"I never heard of tobacco poisoning," Smart said.

"I have," Mrs. Smart said. "Oh, my gosh, Homer. What are we going to do?"

Mason looked at Smart. He could see him, but his features were out of focus, and there was something moving just above his head. It was like a play of light and shadow — or a cloud of smoke. It became a swarm of bees. They swarmed silently around and around and around. "Leroy," Mason said, I think you better drive us in to the doctor."

The medical needs of Caney Valley residents are served by a middle-aged general practitioner whom I'll call Francis Craig and a young associate whom I'll call Henry Rathbone. These two physicians operate a clinic at Church Hill, a roadside village about midway between Kingsport and the Mason farm, and it was there that Smart drove his wife and son and the Masons. They arrived at the clinic at two o'clock.

"I was alone that afternoon," Dr. Rathbone says. "Dr. Craig was in Kingsport at the hospital — the Holston Valley Community Hospital — making rounds. Lucy, our nurse, called me on the interoffice phone and said that five people had just come in from Caney Valley. Three of them, she said, were acting very strange. She sounded rather agitated. I was with a patient, but I finished up as quickly as I could. Lucy isn't a flighty girl. I went out to the waiting room — and she was entirely correct. They were acting very strange indeed. The women were twitching and jerking and moaning, and one of the men — Mason, it turned out to be — was waving his arms and talking a wild blue streak of gibberish. I thought for a minute that he was simply scared. But then I looked again. He was peering into space and making grabs at the air, and I realized that scared wasn't it at all. He was hallucinating. The other man, the man named Smart, came up and introduced himself and told me what he could about the matter. I gathered that his wife and Mason had been taken right after eating. Then, a little later, Mrs. Mason took sick. Smart and his little boy, however, were perfectly all right. The symptoms, as I made them out, were vertigo, blurred vision, dry mouth, generalized weakness, nausea, and — in Mason's case, at any rate — hallucinations. Smart added that his wife and the Masons had spent the morning stripping tobacco. He wondered if the tobacoo could in some way have poisoned them. I told him no on that. Tobacco poisoning could be only nicotine poisoning, and that couldn't happen from that kind of superficial contact. But they had almost certainly been poisoned. My guess was food poisoning — food intoxication. And, to judge from those clearly central-nervous-system symptoms, it was something pretty serious.

"Smart helped me get his wife and the Masons into the examining room. Mason really needed help. He couldn't even stand alone. We got him stretched out on a cot and as comfortable as possible, and settled the two women in chairs. The blurred vision they all complained of was easy to understand. They all had widely dilated pupils — very glassy-looking. The immediate problem as far as Mason and Mrs. Smart were concerned was nausea. They were sick as dogs, and, to make matters worse, they both had an insatiable thirst. I gave them each an intramuscular injection of trimethobenzamide hydrochloride. That seemed to help the nausea a bit, but it was obvious that they were getting sicker by the minute. Mason was so wild it was hard to keep him from falling off the cot. He kept reaching for imaginary doorknobs, as if he wanted to get out of the room. Sometimes he would be fighting off a swarm of bugs. Then at times he seemed to calm down, and he would point across the room or up at the ceiling and say something about all the beautiful flowers. But most of the time nothing he said made any kind of sense. And Mrs. Smart was almost as bad. She was beginning to hallucinate, too, and raving and thrashing around in her chair. It was unnerving. I really didn't know what to think. Or, rather, there was only one thing I could think of, and that possibility was almost too frightening to contemplate. I mean botulism. Botulism, as you probably know, is the most dangerous of the bacterial food poisonings. It has a mortality rate of about sixty-five percent. It is also, of course, a pretty rare bird. But it happens. As a matter of fact, it had happened right here in eastern Tennessee — in Knoxville — only a couple of weeks before. You probably read about it in the paper. There were seven cases in the outbreak, and two of them were fatal. So botulism was more or less on my mind. I didn't have far to reach. I thought of it the minute I saw those central-nervous-system symptoms.

"I don't mean to say I was certain. Not at all. There were several points that didn't quite fit a diagnosis of botulism. The onset, for one thing, seemed a little too sudden. And the symptoms were not exactly right. The central-nervous-system symptoms that Mrs. Smart and Mason had were more pronounced — more violent — than the central-nervous-system symptoms that are classically characteristic of botulism. But they were close enough. They were certainly too close to ignore. Botulism can be treated, you know. There's an anti-toxin, and if it's given in time it can make all the difference. Dr. Craig agreed with me. I called him at the hospital and gave him the facts and asked him what he thought, and he wasn't for taking any chances, either. He proposed that I call the ambulance service and get them right into the hospital. I was glad to take his advice."

Mason and Mrs. Smart were carried into the emergency room of the Holston Valley Community Hospital in Kingsport at five minutes after four. Mrs. Mason arrived at four-fifteen with Smart and his little boy. They were received by Dr. Craig and (such was his aversion to taking any chances) three hurriedly recruited consultants — a neurosurgeon; the hospital pathologist, Dr. William Harrison; and an internist whom I'll call Richard Johnson. Both Mason and Mrs. Smart were now wildly delirious and almost totally helpless. They were also deeply flushed, dry of mouth, and tormented by an unquenchable thirst, and Mason was shaken by frequent muscle spasms. Mrs. Mason, however, was still only weak,

dry-mouthed, and vertiginous. The emergency-room examination was diagnostically uninstructive. Mason's pulse rate
was a hundred, or about thirty beats faster than normal for a
man, and Mrs. Smart's was eighty-eight, or only slightly
faster than normal for a woman, and both had a temperature
of ninety-nine degrees. Mrs. Mason had no fever, and her
pulse rate was normal. All three had widely dilated pupils
that reacted sluggishly to light. The results of the other routine tests — blood pressure, blood count, urinalysis — were
normal in all three cases.

"I think we were all inclined to accept Dr. Rathbone's first
impression," Dr. Johnson, the internist, says. "The trouble
was obviously some kind of poisoning. What kind was hard
to say. It looked like botulism, and yet it didn't. Hallucinations and disorientation very seldom occur in botulism, and
when they do, they tend to be rather late-developing symptoms. Still, it wasn't a possibility that any of us were willing
to rule out of the picture entirely. Even a hint of botulism is
unsettling. We were standing there in the emergency room
and feeling very unsettled when Smart got up from where
he was sitting with his son and came over. He said his little
boy was complaining about his eyes. Everything looked
funny, Buddy said. That sounded like what had happened to
his wife and the others, so he thought we ought to know.
Also, Smart said, he wasn't feeling too good himself. His
eyes were all right, but he had a cramping pain in his stomach, and he was beginning to feel a little nauseated. Well,
that decided us. Botulism antitoxin isn't something you can
get at any drugstore. Or at any hospital, for that matter.
There isn't that much demand for it. The nearest possible
source we could think of was the Poison Control Center at

the University of Tennessee Memorial Hospital, in Knoxville. Robert Lash, the director of the Center, had laid in a supply of antitoxin during the botulism outbreak they had over there earlier in the month, and maybe some of it was left. I went to the phone and gave Dr. Lash a ring, and we were in luck. He still had several hundred thousand units on hand. He said he would get it off at once by a special highway-patrol messenger. It was now about a quarter to five. We should have it by seven o'clock."

It took Dr. Lash about ten minutes to arrange with his dispensary and the Tennessee highway patrol for the dispatch of some five hundred thousand units of polyvalent botulinus antitoxin to the Holston Valley Community Hospital. He then returned to his desk and put in a call to Nashville — to Cecil B. Tucker, director of the Division of Preventable Diseases of the Tennessee State Department of Public Health, in the Cordell Hull State Office Building there. Botulism is a communicable disease, and consequently a notifiable one. In Tennessee, as in all other states, its appearance (proved or suspected) must be reported to the state health authorities for prompt investigation. When Dr. Tucker came on the line, Dr. Lash gave him the required report.

"I wasn't as startled as I might have been by that call from Dr. Lash," Dr. Tucker says. "Botulism was no great novelty in Tennessee that month, you know. My only thought was something like 'Here we go again.' I thanked him and hung up and put in a call to Kingsport — to Dr. Johnson. I wanted a few more facts before sending an investigator up there. But I had Dan Jones standing by. Dr. Jones is an Epidemic Intelligence Service officer assigned to us by the U.S. Public

Health Service through its Communicable Disease Center, in Atlanta. I got Dr. Johnson, and he described the cases. He gave me the clinical picture and what he could of the epidemiology, and I began to have my doubts. It just didn't sound like botulism. But that, of course, was only an opinion. Botulism was still a possibility, so we had to go and see. I told Dr. Johnson that Dr. Jones would be up there in the morning, and started to say goodbye. And Dr. Johnson said, 'Wait a minute.' I waited. Then Dr. Johnson came back on. 'By the way,' he said. 'One of the doctors here has been talking to one of the patients, and he says he just mentioned something about eating Jimson weed.' I don't remember what I said to that. Except that I would call him back.

"Dr. Jones had heard what I heard. He was listening in on an extension. We lit out down the hall and up the stairs to the chemical lab. That's where we keep our file on poisons. I pulled out the card on Jimson-weed poisoning, and no wonder I'd had my doubts. I'll read you what it says under 'Symptoms and Findings': 'Pupils dilated, dry burning sensation of mouth, thirst, difficulty in swallowing, fever, generalized flushing, headache, nausea, excitement, confusion, delirium, rapid pulse and respiration, urinary retention, convulsions.' It was almost word for word the clinical picture that Dr. Johnson had given me on the two patients more seriously stricken. We went back downstairs to my office. I got Dr. Johnson on the phone again and told him what we had found. I said it very much looked to me as though Jimson-weed poisoning was the answer to his problem. Dr. Johnson said he thought I was right. They had done some checking themselves, he said, and they had come to that same conclusion."

266

Jimson weed (or stinkweed, or thorn apple, or devil's-trumpet) is a big, hardy, cosmopolitan annual of Asian origin. It is known to science as *Datura stramonium* and is a member of the large and generally noxious Solanaceae, or nightshade, family of plants. Other members of this family include tobacco, horse nettle, henbane, belladonna, the petunia, the tomato, and the Irish potato. All these plants, including the tomato and the potato, are at least in some respects pernicious. Jimson weed is entirely so. Its leaves, its seeds, its flowers, and its roots all contain a toxic alkaloid called hyoscyamine. Hyoscyamine is closely related to atropine and is, if anything, more toxic. Jimson weed is distributed throughout most of the United States. It made its first appearance here in the early seventeenth century, possibly as early as 1607. Some authorities think it may have been introduced in ballast and other rubbish discharged from the ships that landed Captain John Smith and his fellow Virginia colonists at Jamestown in that year. In any event, it seems reasonably certain that it entered this country there. Early records indicate that the Powhatan Indians of coastal Virginia called it the "white man's weed." The white colonists of Virginia and elsewhere, on the other hand, called it "Jamestown weed." Robert Beverly refers to it as Jamestown weed in his *History and Present State of Virginia*, of 1705, and gives a recognizable, if somewhat excessive, depiction of its hallucinatory powers:

This being an early Plant, was gather'd very young for a boil'd salad by some of the Soldiers . . . and some of them ate plentifully of it, the Effect of which was a very pleasant Comedy; for they turn'd natural Fools upon it for several Days. One would blow a Feather in the Air; another would dart Straws at it with much Fury; and another stark naked was sitting up in a Corner, like a

Monkey grinning and making Mows at them; a Fourth would fondly kiss and paw his Companions, and snear in their Faces, with a Countenance more antik than any in a Dutch Droll. In this frantik Condition they were confined, lest they in their Folly should destroy themselves; though it was observed that all their Actions were full of Innocence and Good Nature. Indeed, they were not very cleanly; for they would have wallow'd in their own Excrements, if they had not been prevented. A Thousand such simple Tricks they play'd, and after Eleven Days, return'd themselves again, not remembering anything that had pass'd.

The other names by which Jimson weed — which is, of course, a corruption of "Jamestown weed" — is sometimes known are more conventionally descriptive. They call attention to one or another of its several notable characteristics. The plant gives off a fetid smell; its fruit, or seed pod, is barbed with thorns, like a chestnut bur; and its poisonous flowers — milky white and sometimes streaked with purple — are trumpet-shaped. Jimson weed is in every sense a weed. Like beggar's-lice and tumbleweed and the cocklebur, it flourishes almost everywhere and is everywhere detested. It sprouts early (as Beverly noted), it grows fast, and it blooms until late in the fall. Its size, for an annual, is considerable. It often reaches a height of six feet, and it averages around four. Like most other successful weeds, Jimson weed can exist on even the poorest land, but its existence there is no more than dogged survival. It does well only in fertile soil, and when it finds itself so placed it feeds voraciously — as voraciously, and as destructively, as corn or cotton. It is also, however, among the easiest of weeds to control. A couple of swipes with a scythe or a hoe before the seeds are formed will clear the most firmly established Jimson-weed jungle. Its presence on cropland or in pasture is thus traditionally taken as a sign of indifferent farming. Mark Twain was aware of its reputation, and in *Tom Sawyer* he turned it to effective atmospheric use: "She [Aunt Polly] went to the open door and stood in it and looked out among the tomato vines and 'jimpson' weeds that constituted the garden." Livestock are repelled by its smell, which is so rank that only animals addled by hunger are rash enough to ignore it. Jimson-weed poisoning in livestock is almost entirely limited to the ingestion of hay or ensilage accidentally contaminated with Jimson-weed seeds or leaves, and such cases are relatively few. Man is less instinctively prudent. Most people find the smell of Jimson weed repellent, but it frequently fails to repel them. Jimson-weed poisoning in man, though hardly commonplace, is anything but rare. "During the past five years at the University of Virginia Hospital, which services a large southern rural area, *Datura* has accounted for approximately four percent of pediatric patients admitted because of ingestion of a toxic substance," Joe E. Mitchell and Fred N. Mitchell, both members of the Department of Pediatrics of the University of Virginia School of Medicine, reported to the *Journal of Pediatrics* in 1955. "Although distinctly less frequent than kerosene or salicylate intoxication, *Datura* has had about the same incidence as lead, barbiturates, alcohol, rodenticides, and insecticides as a source of poisoning." Jimson-weed poisoning in children can usually be laid to innocence. The seeds are mistaken for nuts, or are used in play as "pills." Its adult victims are more variously poisoned. Some of them are victims of homespun credulity (folk medicine recommends a tea of Jimson-weed leaves for the relief of asthma, constipation, and certain other ills), and some are victims of a credulous sophistication (the street-corner pharmacopoeia recommends Jimson-weed seeds for a liberating hallucinatory experience). A few of them — including, as it turned out, Homer Mason and his family — are victims of simple ignorance.

The doctor to whom one of the patients in the emergency room of the Holston Valley Community Hospital that October afternoon in 1963 said "something about eating Jimson weed" was William Harrison, the hospital pathologist, and the patient was Leroy Smart. That wasn't, however, exactly what he said.

"I'd been talking to Smart about the meal he had fixed that noon," Dr. Harrison says. "I wanted to know just what had been eaten and just how it had been prepared. It bothered me. I don't mean I had any ideas. It was only that Mason and Mrs. Smart had taken sick almost immediately after eating. That was a little suspicious. Either that or a rather odd coincidence. But the trouble was, of course, that ordinary bacterial food poisoning doesn't act that way. It doesn't come on that fast. It takes hours, and even days. The same is true of most other kinds of food poisoning. About the only poisons that hit in a matter of minutes are chemical poisons, like antimony and sodium fluoride, and the symptoms they produce are nothing like those we had here. So I was simply floundering. But something I said must have struck a chord in Smart. His whole expression changed. Come to think of it, he said, there was something he hadn't thought to mention about that meal — something a little unusual. The tomatoes they'd had weren't ordinary tomatoes. They were grafts. They were grown on a tomato stalk that Mason had grafted onto a Jimson-weed plant. He wondered if that might have had anything to do with the trouble.

"That was when I spoke to Dr. Johnson. I knew he was talking to Nashville, and I thought they ought to know. The way he heard it was a little confused. Or maybe I was a little confusing. I probably was. I mean, I knew without any question that Jimson weed was the answer. It answered all our questions — the central-nervous-system symptoms, the sudden onset after eating, everything. But the whole thing was so fantastic. It was also such a relief. Jimson-weed poisoning can be extremely serious. It can be fatal. Still, almost anything is preferable to botulism. And not only that. It relieved our minds about Smart and his little boy. The late onset of their symptoms suggested a mild exposure. The same was largely true in the case of Mrs. Mason. Her symptoms were somewhat delayed, and they were also relatively mild. In fact, in the end we didn't even admit those three to the hospital. It was different, of course, with Mason and Mrs. Smart. They were really sick. They didn't seem to be in critical condition, but they certainly needed hospitalization. We put them to bed and started them on a course of oral pilocarpine, a nerve stimulant that would serve to counteract the action of the toxin on their vision by stimulating the parasympathetic nerves. But that was about all we could do for them. There is no specific treatment for Jimson-weed poisoning.

"I had another talk with Smart just before he left the hospital. I had no real connection with the case, of course, but I was interested — intensely interested. Smart was with his son and Mrs. Mason. Dr. Craig had given her ten milligrams of pilocarpine for symptomatic relief, and she seemed to be in pretty good shape. I was particularly interested in the nature of the tomato graft. Smart couldn't help me on that. He said I'd have to talk to Mason, since Mason did all the gardening. He was able to tell me the why of it, though. It was really a bright idea. Mistaken, to be sure, but most ingenious. Mason wanted a hardy, frost-resistant tomato — one that would ripen late in the fall. And he knew that Jimson weed was a hardy, frost-resistant plant that flourished until well into November. So he put the two together. He was right, too. The graft was completely successful. As a matter of fact, Smart said, that tomato they ate at dinner was the very first fruit of the experiment. It had only that morning turned ripe enough to pick. It was a good-sized, good-looking tomato, he said, and it had a good flavor. It tasted like any good home-grown, vine-ripened tomato. He had eaten one slice, and so had his wife and Mrs. Mason. It was possible that his wife's slice had been one of the big center slices. His own had been an end slice, and Buddy's had been only a sliver. Mason, on the other hand, had eaten three or four slices.

"I looked in on Mason the following morning. He was still sick, still flat on his back, but he seemed to be perfectly rational. Except, I should say, on the subject of his tomatoes. He knew what had happened. Somebody on the staff had already told him the cause of the family outbreak. But he didn't quite believe it. He had never heard of Jimson-weed poisoning. Jimson weed was a weed like any other weed to him. I didn't argue with him. We just talked, and I finally got him around to telling me about his grafting technique. The Jimson-weed plant he had used was growing in a fence row not far from his house. He made the graft at the first fork of a secondary branch, snipping off the branch and inserting the sharpened stem of a tomato plant into the pithy center of the stump. Then he fastened the parts together with a clothespin until the union healed. And that was all there was to it. It was simplicity itself. I was really quite impressed, and I told him so. I asked him how he happened to get the idea. He looked a little surprised. What idea? The idea of grafting tomatoes? Why, that wasn't his idea. He got it from a friend — a fellow over in the next valley. I'll give him the name of Clayton. Clayton had been growing tomatoes on Jimson-weed grafts for years. He was always fooling around with plants.

"Well, that was an interesting piece of news. It was flabbergasting. And it raised some flabbergasting questions. Why hadn't we heard of this before? Or had Clayton never been poisoned? And if he hadn't been poisoned, why not? And so on. It was some little time before we got any answers. By 'we' I mean the State Health Department, the Hawkins County Health Department, and the interested doctors here at the hospital. The first step was one that would have been taken in any case. Somebody from the county went out to Mason's farm and got a sample Jimson-weed tomato and sent it in to Nashville for analysis. Then Clayton was interviewed. He confirmed what Mason had said. He and his family had been growing and eating Jimson-weed tomatoes for years — since 1958, to be exact. No, he never sold any. There were only enough for home use. They ate them raw, they ate them stewed, and they ate them canned. And without any ill effects. The very idea that they might be poisonous astonished him. He, too, had never heard of Jimson-weed poisoning. As it happened, he hadn't yet sampled this year's crop of Jimson-weed tomatoes, but he was glad to give the investigator a couple for analysis.

"We got the report from the laboratory sometime the following week. It made rather curious reading. It raised as many questions as it answered. It fully confirmed the cause of the Mason family's outbreak. They were victims of Jimson-weed poisoning. There are no exact data on the toxicity of hyoscyamine, the principal stramonium alkaloid. It is known, however, that hyoscyamine is somewhat more toxic than atropine, and that as little as two milligrams of atropine will produce such symptoms as rapid pulse, dryness of the mouth, pupil dilation, and blurred vision. Well, the Mason tomato yielded 4.2 milligrams of stramonium alkaloid per hundred grams of tomato. That worked out to 6.36 milligrams of alkaloid for the whole tomato. In other words, it was very definitely toxic. But the Clayton tomatoes were different. They averaged just 1.9 milligrams per hundred grams of tomato. Or a scant three milligrams for the whole. I couldn't understand it. None of us could. Why should Mason's Jimson-weed tomatoes be twice as toxic as Clayton's? Why should there be any difference at all? That was one question. And how was it that the Claytons could eat their tomatoes with impunity? That was another question. The toxic content of the Clayton tomatoes wasn't very high, but it was far from negligible. There must surely have been times when Clayton and his wife each ate a whole tomato, and three milligrams of hyoscyamine is quite enough to cause trouble.

"I think I can say that we found the answer to one of those questions. I can also say, I think, that I helped to find it although I certainly didn't realize it at the time. I picked up a

274

piece of information, but I didn't know what it meant. It had to do with grafting. A few days after the laboratory report came in, I had another talk with Mason. I drove down to his farm. Both he and Mrs. Smart were home by then and fully recovered, and he took me out and showed me his Jimson-weed tomato plant. It was quite a sight — a tomato plant growing out of a big, bushy Jimson weed. I even took some pictures of it. On the way home, I dropped in on Clayton. I introduced myself and told him of my interest in the case, and we discussed it for a while. Then he showed me *his* Jimson-weed tomato patch. It didn't look much like Mason's. It seemed to be all tomato plants. They were growing out of Jimson-weed stock, but the Jimson-weed branches were practically bare. Only the tomato plants were lush and leafy. I spoke to Clayton about that, and told him how Mason's plants looked. Clayton shrugged. This was the way he did it, he said. He liked to keep the Jimson weed pretty well pruned of leaves in order to concentrate the growth in the tomato plant. He didn't know why Mason didn't do the same.

"I thought that was an interesting point. As I say, I didn't know what it meant. I didn't know if it had any significance at all. But I passed the information on to Dan Jones at the State Health Department in Nashville. He was handling the case at that end, and he was as fascinated, and as puzzled, by it as I was. And that was as far as my contribution went. Dr. Jones took it from there. I understand he read everything he could find on Jimson weed in the hope of making some sense out of the case. Finally, he wrote to an expert on *Datura stramonium* — a professor of botany at Columbia University named Ray F. Dawson. Dr. Jones and I had both been under the impression that the alkaloid in Jimson weed was produced only in the roots of the plant and then distributed to the stem, the leaves, and the fruit. Dr. Dawson straightened us out on that. That was his contribution. The way he explained it to Dr. Jones, Clayton's pruning trick made a considerable difference. Hyoscyamine is synthesized also in the *leaves* of a Jimson-weed plant. So Mason could hardly have grown a more toxic tomato if that had been his aim.

"The other question is still unanswered. We don't know how Clayton could have eaten his tomatoes with impunity, and I doubt if we ever will. There are certain facts that may have some bearing on the matter. Different Jimson-weed plants produce somewhat different amounts of stramonium alkaloid. It depends on where and how they grow. And people differ somewhat in their sensitivity to the alkaloid. But that doesn't take us very far. I'm afraid it doesn't take us anywhere at all."